THE STUDY OF ANATOMY IN BRITAIN,
1700–1900

The Body, Gender and Culture

Series Editor: Lynn Botelho

Titles in this Series

1 Courtly Indian Women in Late Imperial India
Angma Dey Jhala

2 Paracelsus's Theory of Embodiment: Conception and Gestation in
Early Modern Europe
Amy Eisen Cislo

3 The Prostitute's Body: Rewriting Prostitution in Victorian Britain
Nina Attwood

4 Old Age and Disease in Early Modern Medicine
Daniel Schäfer

5 The Life of Madame Necker: Sin, Redemption and the Parisian Salon
Sonja Boon

6 Stays and Body Image in London: The Staymaking Trade, 1680–1810
Lynn Sorge-English

7 Prostitution and Eighteenth-Century Culture: Sex, Commerce and Morality
Ann Lewis and Markman Ellis (eds)

8 The Aboriginal Male in the Enlightenment World
Shino Konishi

9 Anatomy and the Organization of Knowledge, 1500–1850
Matthew Landers and Brian Muñoz (eds)

10 Blake, Gender and Culture
Helen P. Bruder and Tristanne J. Connolly (eds)

11 Age and Identity in Eighteenth-Century England
Helen Yallop

12 The Politics of Reproduction in Ottoman Society, 1838–1900
Gülhan Balsoy

FORTHCOMING TITLES

Interpreting Sexual Violence, 1660–1800
Anne Greenfield (ed.)

Women, Agency and the Law, 1300–1700
Bronach Kane and Fiona Williamson (eds)

Sex, Identity and Hermaphrodites in Iberia, 1500–1800
Richard Cleminson and Francisco Vázquez García

The English Execution Narrative, 1200–1700
Katherine Royer

British Masculinity and the YMCA, 1844–1914
Geoff Spurr

THE STUDY OF ANATOMY IN BRITAIN, 1700–1900

BY

Fiona Hutton

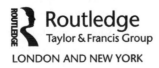
Routledge
Taylor & Francis Group

LONDON AND NEW YORK

First published 2013 by Pickering & Chatto (Publishers) Limited

Published 2016 by Routledge
2 Park Square, Milton Park, Abingdon, Oxfordshire OX14 4RN
711 Third Avenue, New York, NY 10017, USA

First issued in paperback 2015

Routledge is an imprint of the Taylor & Francis Group, an informa business

BRITISH LIBRARY CATALOGUING IN PUBLICATION DATA

Hutton, Fiona, 1969– author.
The study of anatomy in Britain, 1700–1900. – (The body, gender and culture)
1. Human anatomy – Study and teaching – England – Manchester – History
– 18th century. 2. Human anatomy – Study and teaching – England – Oxford
– History – 18th century. 3. Human anatomy – Study and teaching – England –
Manchester – History – 19th century. 4. Human anatomy – Study and teaching
– England – Oxford – History – 19th century. 5. Human dissection – England –
Manchester – History – 18th century. 6. Human dissection – England – Oxford
– History – 18th century. 7. Human dissection – England – Manchester – History – 19th century. 8. Human dissection – England – Oxford – History – 19th
century. 9. Dead bodies (Law) – Great Britain.
I. Title II. Series
611'.00711'42-dc23

ISBN-13: 978-1-138-66479-1 (pbk)
ISBN-13: 978-1-8489-3421-4 (hbk)
Typeset by Pickering & Chatto (Publishers) Limited

CONTENTS

Acknowledgements   ix

Introduction   1
1 Medical Education in Oxford and Manchester before the 1832
    Anatomy Act   15
2 Dissection in Oxford and Manchester: Supply and Demand before
    1832   43
3 The Anatomy Act and the Poor   71
4 The Working of the Anatomy Act in Oxford and Manchester   89
5 Medical Education in Oxford and Manchester after the Anatomy Act   111
6 Some Contemporary Parallels   131
Conclusion   139
Appendix   143

Notes   165
Works Cited   187
Index   199

ACKNOWLEDGEMENTS

This book started out as a thesis submitted to Oxford Brookes University. I am grateful to the university for the studentship which allowed its completion and to my supervisors, Jonathan Andrews and Professor Steve King.

I would like to thank the staff of the Oxfordshire Record Office, the Centre for Oxfordshire Studies, the Bodleian Library, the Central Reference Library in Manchester, the John Rylands Library at the University of Manchester, the National Archives and the Royal College of Surgeons. In particular I am grateful to Judith Curthoys, Keeper of the Christ Church College Archives, Elizabeth Boardman, Keeper of the Radcliffe Infirmary Records, and Rini Banerjee of the Manchester Royal Infirmary for allowing me much time to examine papers not generally available to the public. Thanks also go to the people who gave their time to discuss aspects of the work or provide valuable references: Richard Dyson, Bill White, Julian Read, Mark Steadman, Sam Alberti, Ian Roberts and Rob Newton. I am especially grateful to Helen MacDonald for sharing her work with me and for her support of this book, and to my editor, Ruth Ireland at Pickering & Chatto, and to her predecessor, Daire Carr, who encouraged me to continue with the work at a particularly difficult time.

An earlier version of Chapter 4 appeared as 'The Working of the 1832 Anatomy Act in Oxford and Manchester' in *Family and Community History*, 9 (2006), pp. 125–39.

I dedicate the work to Ian Roberts and our children, Joe and Ben.

INTRODUCTION

The 1832 Anatomy Act had been largely ignored within the field of medical history until the groundbreaking work of Ruth Richardson.[1] Richardson is largely credited with 'rediscovering' the Act in 1988, yet despite her assertion that there was much to add to her work, there have been surprisingly few further studies in the succeeding twenty-five years dealing with the passing and impact of the Act, particularly within a regional context. This book examines the impact of the 1832 Anatomy Act on the study of anatomy within two very different regions and institutions. The choice of Manchester and Oxford provides a contrast between a new and ambitious provincial centre with arguably the first fully organized provincial medical school and a highly traditional centre for medical training based on university education.

An examination of the working of the Anatomy Act illuminates the supply of bodies which was vital for the study of anatomy, a discipline that was becoming the lynchpin of surgical training from the eighteenth century. An intimate understanding of anatomy and skill in dissection were considered to be important components in the education of surgeons, and then of all medical men, and was central to their claim for professional status. Anatomy became the dominant discipline in medical education in the nineteenth century. This work questions the rising role of anatomy in the training of doctors and then investigates whether the claims of legislators and civil servants of an increased supply of cadavers, and therefore attendant benefits for medical education, were justified. More specifically, against the broader background of the comparative and contrasting roles of Oxford and Manchester in early nineteenth-century medical training, this work seeks to determine whether the Anatomy Act was a key factor in the decline and ultimate demise of the independent medical schools in these regions, and to assess how successful local surgeons were in claiming bodies from workhouses and other public institutions.

The application of the Anatomy Act provides an alternative insight into attitudes to the poor by the ruling elite and wider middle class at the start of the nineteenth century. The book delineates the impact of the Anatomy Act on the poor and its relationship with the subsequent Poor Law Amendment Act in Oxford and Manchester, taking the analysis well beyond the confines of the metropolitan conurbation. It has been necessary to examine the perception and reality of the threat of dissection on the poor, especially those at risk of dying in the workhouse and the hospital, and how this was manifested. The Act allows us a limited means to examine feelings about the dead body and its place in religious observance and the role of funeral ritual for all classes.

Ruth Richardson's highly influential book *Death, Dissection and the Destitute* is the major work analysing the Act from inception through to legislation and its subsequent impact on the poor and their death beliefs. Richardson's approach was to examine the effect of the legislation upon the poor, and Tim Marshall viewed *Death, Dissection and the Destitute* as 'an essential supplement to Thompson's *The Making of the English Working Class*'.[2] This was overstating the case. In spite of the extensive nature of Richardson's account, she herself conceded that it left much undone and focused almost completely on London. She called for more detailed regional and international studies on the implications of the Anatomy Act and remained largely unconcerned with medical education. There has been work on nineteenth-century bodysnatching, dissection and anatomy in the United States and Canada,[3] while Helen Macdonald's recent work examines the cadaver trade in London, Edinburgh and beyond to Australia and is an extremely interesting addition to the historiography.[4] Yet there has been a limited number of local British studies, and the present work adds to the collection by comparing two regional centres with very different philosophies of medical education.[5]

Before analysing the impact of the Anatomy Act, it will be necessary to examine the nature of anatomical training in eighteenth- and nineteenth-century England. The Act became desirable only after traditional sources of cadavers became compromised and inadequate to satisfy a growing need for improved anatomical skill.

Bodysnatching and Dissection

One notable development of consumer society in the eighteenth and nineteenth centuries was a greater demand from an increasingly wealthy middle class able and willing to pay for more assured medical care from expert practitioners, particularly in the area of surgery. Doctors themselves, and surgeons in particular, were anxious to distance themselves from the growing number of 'quacks' in the unregulated medical marketplace. Claims to scientific expertise based on anatomy and dissection were a means of detaching the proficient and educated from the charlatan. It was increasingly believed that successful surgeons had to be skilled and fast, which produced an emphasis on anatomy and dissection in medical education, with a corresponding increase in demands for cadavers. Large numbers of bodies were needed in part because methods of preservation were inadequate until late in the nineteenth century. These demands for bodies were initially met by the practice of bodysnatching until the Anatomy Act was passed in 1832.

Prior to 1832 the only legal source of bodies for anatomists was the very few murderers executed in Britain, who had dissection added to their sentences from 1752. This was 'an added humiliation' as these criminals were denied the 'meticulous attention to the proper forms of burial ... required to ensure the peaceful departure of the dead'.[6] This source became increasingly inadequate in light of the growing number of medical students and led to the rise of bodysnatching, which was of course common to all social classes. Astley Cooper (1768–1841),[7] the elite London surgeon, boasted of his ability to procure any corpse in England, yet the poor were disproportionately at risk from the 'resurrection men' due to their obvious inability to pay for secure coffins, superior burial sites and well-rewarded watchmen.

What started as a handful of men, often medical students, supplying a limited number of anatomists grew from the early 1800s into a huge and lucrative trade with national transportation of cadavers. The development of this trade led to greater vigilance by the general public and therefore increasing shortages and attendant inflation in body prices. There is much evidence of a trade in bodies centred on Manchester, supplying Edinburgh and London, and this is examined in Chapter 2, where the growth of anatomy in Manchester and Oxford prior to the Anatomy Act is described. Manchester appears to have been a centre of much anatomy and dissection activity, starting within the Literary and Philosophical Society in the late 1700s and developing into several successful private anatomy schools. There are great difficulties in tracing the extent of such covert supply as the investigation is dependent upon finding relevant newspaper coverage and comments in private papers. As a result the analysis can only ever outline minimum levels of body supply.

Oxford Medical School was an early centre of anatomy in the seventeenth century, but by the time the Anatomy School was built at the end of the century, the supply of bodies was difficult. The seventeenth-century Oxford anatomists seem to have had some limited opportunity to dissect from deaths within their own coterie of scholars and private patients. This is a particularly interesting aspect of seventeenth-century dissection, where, certainly in Oxford, there seems to have been less antagonism to dissection than in the later period, and this is examined in Chapter 1. Public attitudes may have hardened after the 1752 Murder Act, particularly as demands for greater numbers of bodies became more obvious. Oxford University never succeeded in establishing a reliable source of bodies in the nineteenth century and had to depend on the occasional body from the London trade, and it was hopeful of the Anatomy Act rectifying this dearth. I can find only one instance of a group of Oxfordshire bodysnatchers appearing at the Oxford Assizes, and this is outlined in Chapter 2. Again, however, it must be noted that the covert nature of the trade in bodies means that anatomical activities may have been much greater than indicated in surviving records.

The cholera epidemic is a fruitful area for researchers of the Anatomy Act as much of the furore surrounding the bill finds voice in the panic over the epidemic. Sean Burrell and Geoffrey Gill, in their study of cholera in Liverpool, noted that the riots during the height of the disease in the city were the result of fears over bodysnatching, 'burking', the medical profession and dissection. They went further than most historians of cholera and claimed that in the words of George Rudé, 'the English probably stood near to revolution only in 1832'. To Rudé's list of reasons – 'Irish unrest, rural disturbance and popular and middle-class excitement over the first Reform Bill'[8] – Burrell and Gill wished to add dissection, bodysnatching and the cholera epidemic.[9] Manchester, in particular, was the setting for a major cholera riot that was sparked by an unauthorized dissection, and this is covered in detail in Chapter 3. Much of the work on the Anatomy Act pre-dating Richardson examined the Act from the perspective of social order. Chapter 3 examines a lesser-known anatomy riot in neighbouring Sheffield in 1835, first described by F. K. Donnelly.[10] Notably, Donnelly gave illuminating details about the passing of the Act along with examples of working-class reaction well before Richardson's work. Oxford did not experience such disturbances, but there were enclosure riots that appear to have included bodysnatching and anatomy within the rioters' grievances, and is examined in Chapter 2. Unlike Cambridge University, Oxford did not experience a dedicated anatomy riot, but the medical school watched tumultuous events in Cambridge after the passing of the Act with concern. Much of my work has used Cambridge and its university as a point of comparison relating to shortage of bodies. Cambridge experienced shortages but made greater efforts to address this problem in order to develop its medical school. My own research indicates that anatomy was never a key element in public riot, but concern over dissection was an issue in working-class resentment and disquiet when other factors came in to play.

The Anatomy Act and Body Supply

The Anatomy Act of 1832 allowed for the so-called 'unclaimed' bodies of the poor to be removed from workhouses and dissected by doctors at recognized medical schools by licensed anatomists. The term 'unclaimed' referred to bodies that remained within the workhouse forty-eight hours after death. The Anatomy Act never made clear whether claimants of bodies had to be genuine relatives and whether they then became liable for the cost of burial, nor did it state if relatives and friends had to be informed of a death at all. This vague attitude is echoed in present-day scandals over anatomy, and this phenomenon is examined in Chapter

6. The 1832 Act was introduced ostensibly to increase the supply of cadavers and to remove doctors from the taint of bodysnatching, which hindered their claims to middle-class respectability. My research examines the working of the Act in Oxford and Manchester and draws upon Richardson's analysis of its working in London along with MacDonald's, as well as that of Mark Weatherall and Elizabeth Hurren on Cambridge. Oxford, like Cambridge, struggled to obtain bodies, but later in the period anatomists in Cambridge worked to secure a supply and developed a relationship with the local hospital to alleviate the problem. Oxford gave up teaching medical students and attempted to promote a general scientific education, with medical students going to London to complete clinical studies. The decline of the medical school in Oxford was not arrested until the twentieth century.

Many poor law authorities may have been extremely reluctant to give up bodies to the anatomists, although there were exceptions to this within the London medical schools, and again this book aims to evaluate the situation for Manchester and Oxford. In this context, it is also necessary to consider the contention that the elite surgeons of London moved against the independent schools well before the 1832 Anatomy Act by demanding that the College of Surgeons only recognize dissection at certain centres, notably, the major hospital medical schools.[11] This position is certainly true, and the need to 'walk the wards' outlined in legislation and royal college regulation favoured the development of hospital medical schools. It is likely that the birth of the General Medical Council in 1858 ensured that medical education based upon apprenticeship and private anatomy classes gave way to university and hospital medical schools. Yet few historians of medicine have made any sort of detailed study of the anatomy inspectorate records, and while it is necessary to note the attitude of the royal colleges towards private teaching, the problems of body supply after the anatomy legislation were also a factor in the long-term decline of private medical teaching.

The situation in Manchester is less clear, and supplies of cadavers have been traced for each year from 1832 until 1875, giving a picture of periods of both dearth and plenty. These are of course officially recorded bodies, and so this research, as a result, examines only a minimum level of activity. It is in any case unfortunate that the body numbers supplied in the Anatomy Inspectorate records disappear from the 1870s, which is the period that Hurren has argued witnessed a hardening of attitudes among poor law Guardians and a corresponding rise in bodies available to the anatomists.[12] While Weatherall believes that the Cambridge medical school experienced many of the same problems of body acquisition that Oxford had right up until the end of the nineteenth century,[13] Hurren has discovered important new sources and found that Cambridge did manage to procure large numbers of cadavers from new locations, including Manchester.[14] My own research suggests that at the beginning of the twentieth century Oxford was dealing with very small numbers of bodies, some of which came from Reading and Leicester workhouses. The body supply under the Anatomy Act is examined in Chapter 4.

Poor Law

While welfare historians have generally given little, if any, attention to the Anatomy Act, even where they do accord it more significance this has tended to be confined to its contextual relationship with the Poor Law Amendment Act that followed it in 1834. There is an extensive poor law historiography that has certainly illuminated our understanding of Victorian welfare provision and outlined changes in attitudes to the problem of the destitute, and dying, yet it is a historiography that has continued largely to disregard or ignore the Anatomy Act. The Poor Law Amendment Act and its subsequent advisory rulings aimed to dispense with outdoor relief for able-bodied paupers. The poor law Guardians were to assess whether each person was truly impoverished through the workhouse test, which applied the theory of 'less eligibility', where the level of support from the poor law was to be markedly less than that available from labouring. Indoor relief was to be available through the workhouse, with its harsh work regime and deeply unpopular separation of the sexes (and threat of dissection through the provisions of the Anatomy Act).

Richardson believed that the Anatomy Act and the Poor Law Amendment Act can be taken together as an indication of hardening attitudes to the poor in the wake of the Swing Riots and reform agitation and may more generally be associated with the breakdown of traditional patterns of paternalist support.[15] She saw the Act as a socio-moral move against the poor, as the much-feared penalty of dissection for the worst crimes of murder became a penalty for poverty. She was supported in this by John Pickstone, who asserted that 'it is surely no accident that the first evidence of worry over dissection in Manchester occurred about 1818, that the first working-class denigration of the Infirmary came as a sequel to Peterloo, and that the mass rioting against dissection came in 1832'.[16]

Public disturbances certainly took place over the passing of the Anatomy Act. The significance of this social unrest was obscured by the general hostility towards the medical profession as demonstrated during the height of the cholera outbreak, and the attention given to the turbulence created by the concurrent passage of the Reform Bill and other measures of social control. This is illuminated in Roy Porter's book *Bodies Politic* with political cartoons on reform illustrated by scenes of post-mortem examinations.[17] Roland Quinault and John Stevenson have argued convincingly that the global titles given to popular protests such as Luddism and Chartism may have contained many different strands that are difficult to separate. Central government records compound this problem by presenting a coherence that protest movements lacked in reality.[18]

The disturbances in Oxford over enclosure would suggest some support for this position, but ultimately the evidence is scanty. This is a contentious area, but the period between 1800 and 1830 was one of severe social change, particularly within the agricultural regions. Separating out the strands of conviction that led to public disorder is of course an extremely difficult task.

Regrettably much of the public record of the poor law has been destroyed, and what remains rarely record the views of the poor inmates, making it difficult to ascertain any actual fear of anatomization. In Chapters 3 and 4 I attempt an analysis of the pauper view through the remaining records of several unions in the North West and Oxfordshire. Disturbances in workhouses were extremely common, but it has been apparent that few related to the Anatomy Act. Friedrich Engels certainly believed that the Manchester poor would often rather die of starvation than go into the workhouse.[19] Research on Manchester supports the contention that destitution was often preferable to the workhouse, although how much the fear of dissection was a factor is impossible to gauge.

The body supply for Oxford was always difficult after the Anatomy Act. The research undertaken for Manchester suggests that the supply of bodies remained patchy for much of the nineteenth century but became easier at the end of the period, when the city was once again able to supply other parts of the country. There is much evidence to suggest, however, that Manchester poor law Guardians often protected the bodies of the poor dying in the workhouse, preferring to bury them than give them to the anatomists. This is also the case within the Radcliffe Infirmary in Oxford, which is considered in Chapter 4. Again, it is unfortunate that the Anatomy Inspectorate records deteriorate after 1875. There are very few Oxford poor law records in existence, but an approach for bodies was made by the Anatomy School, without success, to a neighbouring union in 1868, suggesting that there was an inadequate supply from the Oxford Union. Again, however, care needs to be taken as the present research can only examine anatomical activity where it was officially recorded, and anatomists often claimed inadequate supplies even when the figures contradict this opinion. The promise made to nineteenth-century doctors about the supply that would be realized after the Anatomy Act was bound to result in a perceived shortage and therefore ultimate disappointment.

Death and the Poor

Prior to the passing of the Anatomy Act, the only legal source of bodies was from the ranks of condemned prisoners, limited solely to murderers from 1752. There is much evidence from Oxford to suggest that prisoners who were to be hanged and their supporters were desperate to avoid anatomization where there were near-riots between the townspeople and the anatomists, and these are examined in Chapter 2. It has also been necessary to examine the rise of private burial companies as a reaction to fear of mass burial and anatomization. Some historians have argued that several private cemetery companies of the nineteenth century recognized fear of the Anatomy Act as a factor in their own aim to inter the poor with as much security as the rich.[20] My own research supports this contention.

I have found little evidence, however, in either Manchester or Oxford to suggest that the Anatomy Act was of particular concern to paupers in the workhouses after 1832, although it was an issue for protest before the passing of the Act, and it must be borne in mind that much of the direct evidence has been destroyed. In both my regional foci there is much evidence that bodies, other than genuinely unknown vagrants, were protected by the poor law authorities. They may, therefore, be noteworthy in this respect.

Medical Education

In the eighteenth century the developing medical profession was characterized by a great divide between the university-educated elite of physicians and the apprenticed surgeons and surgeon-apothecaries, as well as that between the hospital-based specialists and the increasing group of general practitioners. Reform after a period of stagnation became possible in the increasingly centralized and interventionist state of the nineteenth century. Ambitious groups in the medical profession benefited from regulatory legislation, medical education and an increasingly wealthy middle class who were prepared to pay generously for medical claims to expertise.

The growth of an increasingly affluent society during the eighteenth century enabled the emergence of a middle class ready and willing to pay for treatment from an array of supposedly orthodox practitioners as well as the derided 'quacks'. The aftermath of the Age of Enlightenment encouraged doctors to believe that disease could be mastered through increasing medical knowledge, based on anatomy. Alongside this growing confidence, doctors could use the claims of expertise in medicine to distance themselves from unorthodox healers in a very competitive marketplace. This expertise could demonstrate itself in knowledge of the mysteries of the body beneath the skin. Doctors defined themselves through skill in anatomy and dissection. This mastery largely became the province of the surgeon and general practitioner, a class of medical men anxious not only to detach themselves from those less qualified but also to claim their own level of knowledge as distinct from the physician, and to profit from the demand for accessible medical care.

At the end of the eighteenth century there were eighteen organizations issuing generally recognized diplomas, degrees and licences to medical men. The plethora of awarding bodies had little power to proscribe unlicensed practitioners, and doctors of the day had to ply their trade alongside the whole gamut of bonesetters, midwives, druggists and quacks. They could, however, confer status and position on the doctor in the increasingly competitive free market for medical care and alleviate the marginal position of medical men in middle-class society. Expertise in anatomy became one of the means for medical men, physicians and surgeons to gain approved knowledge and thus distance themselves not only from the mass of unorthodox healers but also from the less expert men at the lower end of the profession.

Doctors experienced a growing notion of unity during the nineteenth century and instituted a raft of measures to ensure that they were separated from unqualified and unlicensed practitioners. The 1858 Medical Register was a key component, but other initiatives that need to be accorded significance include the 1815 Apothecaries Act.[21] This Act marked an initial attempt to outline a basic syllabus focused on dissection and standards for the medical practitioner, and it indicated the need for central control of qualifications and practice. By 1850 the great majority of doctors had largely abandoned apprenticeship in favour of the hospital, supplemented by private and hospital courses centred on dissection. Training was increasingly specified and examined by the royal colleges.

The nineteenth century saw a growing importance in the idea of science and laboratory work to the medical student, although few historians have examined the role of dissection in the training of surgeons. Yet during the first quarter of the nineteenth century, 'the body rather than the discursive patient was becoming the real object of medicine'.[22] Respectable access to bodies was vital to trainee doctors to further their claims as men of science. Weaknesses in therapy were masked by advances in pathological anatomy and surgery, which raised the image of doctors as scientists. Additionally, expertise in science was a means for surgeon-apothecaries and general practitioners to raise their status. The Anatomy Act was a key attempt to distance doctors from bodysnatchers by providing a reliable means of receiving bodies without lowering the doctors' own status by snatching bodies or dealing with the resurrection men. Indeed, the reputation of medical students was low partly because of this link in the public imagination. In commercial society, orthodoxy was one means of establishing a niche in an increasingly competitive market.

Susan Lawrence has argued compellingly that anatomists were allowed to conduct their business alongside neighbours who knew of their work but were prepared to ignore it as long as social mores were observed.[23] This certainly seems to be the case in Manchester, with several surgeons operating anatomy schools in residential areas without comment. There was a public outcry only when medical men and bodysnatchers made their activities obvious. Dissections at Oxford took place behind the walls of Christ Church, and the small numbers involved seem to have ensured little opposition from the population, although there were public demonstrations of disapproval at the assizes. These issues are examined in Chapters 2 and 3. Contemporary pathologists and anatomists have discovered the same scenario: public anger and ensuing legislative regulation result from activities that step beyond a set of commonly accepted boundaries. Modern-day parallels are examined in the final chapter.

The professional aspirations of the surgeon-apothecaries were the catalyst for the rise of pathological anatomy in the medical curriculum in the 1830s and the attendant need for cadavers. The nineteenth century saw the dominant position of the pure physician eroded, and surgery rose as the more prestigious branch of medicine by the beginning of the twentieth century. The mastery of anatomy allowed surgeons to rise rapidly up the professional ladder. Christopher Lawrence asserted that over the nineteenth century, 'from being the treatment of last resort surgery was establishing itself as the therapy of choice'.[24] However, the harnessing of science was a useful tool for all branches of medicine to emphasize professional expertise.

My research has made extensive use of contemporary publications regarding the role of anatomy in medical education in the eighteenth and nineteenth centuries and follows the debates in the *Lancet* and the *British Medical Journal*. Contemporary writers elevated the detailed and extended study of anatomy for medical students regardless of speciality. It was considered necessary for the upper-class pure physicians and for the more lowly apothecaries and general practitioners, despite the fact that neither group would be likely to experience an operation that required more than a fairly cursory understanding of anatomy. The rise of anatomy suited doctors' pretensions to scientific respectability but was largely unnecessary for the bulk of the profession. Anatomy, like hospital training, was not perhaps the most useful type of training for the majority who were destined for general practice. The pre-eminent position of anatomy in nineteenth-century medical education ultimately, therefore, damaged English physiology, which became the dominant medical discipline in Europe.

The acceptance of surgery as the key discipline (and therefore the importance of anatomy in medical education and the supply of bodies) was a crucial element in the emerging profession's unity and necessary to claims of expertise and status. The mastery of the human body was a vital factor and was an early source of group cohesion for the surgeons in Manchester. Oxford University lagged behind not only the continent but also other British centres, as it was content to continue to educate the gentlemanly physician and remain opposed to premature specialization.

Oxford University was particularly badly affected in attempts to reform science, and especially medicine, in the 1880s by the Agricultural Revolution, which altered its income. Although this also hurt revenues at Cambridge University, Cambridge had a stronger tradition of science, and more power resided in the central university over the colleges, whereas the colleges at Oxford held power over a relatively weak (and poor) central institution. Cambridge embraced anatomical training and later became a leading centre for the study of physiology, together with University College London. Alongside the nature of the university–college relationship, the people at the head of the respective medical schools were also a key factor. Oxford University did much to join the first ranks of anatomy and physiology after the decline in reputation of Henry Acland and the arrival of John Burdon-Sanderson. These developments are examined in Chapter 5.

The Anatomy Act did nothing to provide better or even cheaper medical training, as it led to the long-term decline of independent medical schools in London due to a shortage of bodies. The teaching hospital became the primary focus for dissection, with corpses supplied by on-site mortuaries, as workhouses and other public institutions could not be forced to give up their bodies and many refused. Linked to this is the fact that the private schools of London disappeared shortly after the establishment of the University of London and the University College Hospital in 1834. The private schools of Manchester certainly survived the Anatomy Act and thrived until much later in the century, but this does appear to be based on the ability of one particular teacher, Thomas Turner, to develop a relationship with the Anatomy Inspector. It was his school that ultimately became the medical school of Owens College and then the Victoria University. Oxford University was unable to secure a decent supply of bodies and fell back on the traditional role of educating the pure physician. These developments are examined in Chapters 4 and 5.

Hospitals and the Body Supply

Body supply was also a problem for some medical schools in the United States, notably for one, located in a small community much like Oxford. In 1810 Harvard Medical School relocated to Boston as bodies were 'utterly unattainable at Cambridge', and there were plans to obtain cadavers from the Boston almshouse.[25] The staff recognized the need to compete or be overshadowed by other institutions with easier access to bodies, and one means to this access, certainly accepted in Europe, was the hospital. This was a situation that Oxford failed to realize. As early as 1714 John Bellers (1654–1725) called for the establishment of hospitals in the university towns, as bodies were practically unobtainable.[26] The establishment of the Radcliffe Infirmary in 1770 did not alleviate this problem.

In the nineteenth century, hospitals, particularly in London, began to lose their original charitable impetus and gradually became centres for the pursuit of education and science, with doctors escalating their control at the expense of the original lay governors. An increasingly assertive medical profession attempted to extend its authority and gradually changed the emphasis within voluntary hospitals towards scientific interest over the traditional moral obligation to the sick poor. There is, however, little evidence to suggest that Oxford and Manchester anatomists had access to bodies in their respective infirmaries until late in the nineteenth century, but the role of the hospital post-mortem in teaching is poorly researched and may have been used by anatomists extensively without the need for documentation.

The role of the hospital post-mortem in terms of the widespread acceptability of the practice in hospitals and how this affected private medical schools needs further research. There is some evidence that dissections could be carried out on poor patients in voluntary hospitals without complaint, which would support the argument that independent medical schools felt disadvantaged in the allocation of bodies after the passing of the Anatomy Act. It seems likely that in the early days of the voluntary hospitals the lay governors saw themselves as protectors of the poor against the clinical interests of the doctors. This situation is likely to have changed over the course of the nineteenth century, with medical men taking more control over the admissions list and the running of the wards and with the growth of more invasive and dangerous procedures particularly associated with the rise of surgery. Mary Fissell suggested that Bristol Infirmary was particularly open to dissection and anatomy:

> Student years filled with anatomy, dissection, and grave-robbing on a scale seemingly unequalled by other educational institutions ... While other hospitals practised anatomy and dissection I doubt that it was inevitably such a strong interest and rite of passage for students.[27]

Moreover, she claimed that the possibilities for what she termed 'post-mortem dissection' 'made Infirmary medicine increasingly repugnant to its patients'.[28]

The records of the Manchester hospitals demonstrated little evidence of post-mortem or dissection rates, and that has been a frustrating aspect of the research undertaken for this book. The Radcliffe Infirmary records, however, were more illuminating, and the minute books of the hospital provide fascinating examples of the lay governors going to some lengths to protect the patients and the corpses of the infirmary. This attitude of patronage was eroded over the nineteenth century to some extent; the evidence is examined in Chapter 4.

Where there was a dearth of pauper bodies, anatomists turned their attention to the hospital and coronial post-mortem. Although the former required consent from relatives, and I have noted examples of resistance to this in Chapters 5 and 6, there was a perceptible difference between whole-body dissection, when remains were often removed and kept by anatomists, and the more limited post-mortem to establish cause of death. Of course there is no way of knowing how extensive routine post-mortems were within the dead house of infirmaries. It is tempting to suggest that anatomists used these examinations as opportunities to teach normal as well as pathological anatomy. This is an area that has been addressed by Mac-Donald with regard to Van Diemen's Land; she contends that 'Tasmanian medical men boasted of the opportunities' for dissection in the public hospitals.[29] In 1867 Dr W. L. Crowther wrote 'that the next (aboriginal person) that should be taken ill is to be forwarded to the General Hospital where I need hardly say she will receive every attention at my hands, particularly post mortem'.[30] More recently, MacDonald has claimed that post-mortem examinations were used extensively in England and Scotland for teaching, and that many of the items in old medical collections came from this source and not from full-body dissections.[31]

The research conducted for this work indicates that while post-mortems were carried out at the Manchester Infirmary and the Radcliffe Infirmary, these were not considered to be good teaching opportunities. The bulk of anatomy continued to be taught at private schools in Manchester until later in the nineteenth century, and the rather tenuous clinical relationship between the University of Oxford and the Radcliffe Infirmary did not improve until very late in the nineteenth century when (in addition to a limited number of on-site post-mortem examinations) a small number of bodies were sent for full dissection to the anatomy school. These issues are discussed in Chapters 4 and 5.

The original sources and historiography need to be treated with particular care when examining dissection. Contemporaries and even historians often appear to use the terms dissection and post-mortem interchangeably or even together. It is difficult to gauge whether these terms are viewed as the same procedure or if, in fact, the post-mortem examination may mean a more limited procedure carried out to discover cause of death. The desire to limit the opening of the body to preserve the feelings of relatives and friends is one discussed in Chapter 5 and is the subject of much concern by the growing number of pathology specialists.

A Note on Specialist Sources

The wide-ranging and comparative nature of the book involves the use of a number of different sources. These have been used both quantitatively and qualitatively. Inevitably the survival, depth and scope of sources in Manchester and Oxford differ in important aspects, though not seriously enough to undermine the comparative framework adopted. Dissection, bodysnatching and purchases of cadavers generate an in-built tendency to source destruction. The same can be said for many of the poor law union records for Oxford and Manchester, although in parts these were extremely useful. Another related source which assisted the research on attitudes to the poor and working-class resentment of anatomy was the relevant cholera archives held at the Central Reference Library in Manchester and at the Bodleian Library and City Record Office in Oxford.

The decline in quality of recording in official records towards the end of the nineteenth century and the closure of one important archive of Manchester letters from the poor because of sudden fragility added to the difficulties. Frustratingly, one other source that at first seemed fruitful – Oxford medical student diaries, which held out the prospect of illuminating the medical student experience of teaching – was very limited in reality.

Of greatest use were the anatomy records held at the National Archives in Kew. A complete inspection of all these extensive official records for Manchester and Oxford was made from 1832 to 1875, after which the records become sparse. The sources of bodies were also illuminated by examining the municipal cemetery records held at Oxford City Archives. The records of the Anatomy School at Oxford in the Archives of Christ Church College and in the Bodleian were of use in researching the teaching of anatomy at Oxford.

There are few records relating to the early anatomy schools of Manchester, so much of the research focused on the Manchester Medical Collection held at the John Rylands University Library. These are unique files of information relating to medical men in the city and contain a valuable anatomical museum catalogue.

1 MEDICAL EDUCATION IN OXFORD AND MANCHESTER BEFORE THE 1832 ANATOMY ACT

This chapter considers the development of medical education from the Renaissance and the resultant importance of anatomical training for European doctors of all types. The contrasting situation in England is examined, specifically the education available in Oxford and Manchester, which offered very different experiences for the medical student. The traditional division between medical and surgical education lasted longer in England than elsewhere in Europe. Theoretically English physicians received a university education, while surgeons and surgeon-apothecaries or general practitioners were trained through an amalgam of apprenticeships and private courses. Oxford had a long tradition of medical education that could be traced from the seventeenth century, when the study of anatomy was temporarily elevated within the university but ultimately failed to find favour with the governing body. The result was a small school that remained devoted to the increasingly moribund pure physician. Medical education in Manchester provided for the growing band of surgeon-general practitioners that came to dominate numbers in the medical establishment.

This chapter then goes on to examine the increasing importance of anatomical study in England and the national debate around the necessity for long and specialized training in minute anatomy for surgeons and also increasingly for physicians. This focus grew out of demands from within the medical profession to regulate the qualification and training of doctors. Despite one prominent argument that the bulk of medical practitioners in the eighteenth and nineteenth centuries would have little use for expertise in dissection, those advocating anatomical proficiency won the debate, as knowledge was an influential method of elevating professional status in the face of a perceived threat from the unqualified. The growing demand for 'scientific' medicine ensured that all medical men would need dissection experience, beyond the level of demonstration. Even physicians had to accept that post-mortem work could illustrate a more precise and universal disease process far more clearly than advocating a disorder specific to the individual.

It will be necessary to trace the broad outlines of the growth of hospital-based education alongside anatomical instruction (and the body supply), which had a profound impact on the ability of both centres to deliver acceptable medical training. Oxford University did not recognize the opportunities available at the Radcliffe Infirmary as a source of clinical and post-mortem material, and thus failed to maintain and increase the body supply; meanwhile Manchester anatomy schools appear to have flourished in the early days of anatomical education, with a good supply of bodies and increasing access to hospital cases and deaths. However, both Oxford and Manchester failed to become major centres for medical education. Later chapters examine the role of the Anatomy Act as a component of this failure.

The dominance of anatomy and ultimately hospital-based medicine in English medical education is traced by reference to contemporary publications and journals that covered the eighteenth-century 'anatomy debate' in much detail. Use is made of one surviving Oxford medical school diary as well as the Radcliffe Infirmary and Manchester Royal Infirmary records and the Manchester Medical Collection.

The Elevation of Anatomy in Medical Education in Europe

Knowledge of anatomy had been an important component in a physician's education since the Renaissance, traditionally through demonstrations in large lecture theatres. The first public autopsies took place in Italy from 1286, conducted on saints and holy bodies or for legal reasons, and were limited in their nature. By 1490 there was a new 'flowering of interest in anatomy', and large theatres were built to conduct much more extensive human dissections, which became university-sponsored four-day exhibitions on criminal bodies.[1] These events attracted hundreds of both medical and lay persons. It was recognized that 'no one can be a good or fully trained doctor unless he is familiar with the anatomy of the human body'.[2] These public anatomies became famous throughout Europe with the publication of *De Humani Corporus Fabrica* (Concerning the Construction of the Human Body) in 1543 by Andreas Vesalius (1514–64). *De Humani* contained beautifully executed and accurate illustrations of extensive dissections. It was a new and more accurate departure from the work of Galen (AD 129–c. 216), whose theories had dominated the medical world since the days of the Roman Empire, but who had been forced to rely on the use of animals as human dissection was restricted.

After Vesalius, the work of Girolamo Fabrici (1533–1619), professor of anatomy at Padua in the late sixteenth century, illustrates the growing conflict in the field of anatomy. Fabrici's interest was in the philosophical principles of anatomy and the glory of the work of the Creator, and his technique was to isolate the organs; he therefore conducted few systematic whole-body dissections to illustrate the workings and connections of the body. This focus instituted a growing division between the 'high style' of public dissection examining the philosophical implications of anatomy and the 'low style' of dissection utilized in private lessons. Most interestingly, this 'high style' of dissection led to a division between professors and students with the latter demanding a return to the Vesalian focus on technical skill and whole-body dissection. This conflict has resonances in eighteenth-century Oxford between the 'high style' dissections of the university and the growing demand for 'low style' private lessons, and this theme is re-visited later in the chapter.

Interest in anatomy continued into the Enlightenment with influential figures such as Hermann Boerhaave (1668–1738), professor of anatomy at Leiden University. Boerhaave rarely conducted full-body dissections but limited himself to finding the cause of death in a more limited autopsy. His innovation lay in his use of clinical histories from hospital patients and tracing symptoms through to post-mortem. European medical men increasingly examined patterns of disease and demanded explanations that were to be found through detailed clinical history and post-mortem. Giovanni Battista Morgagni (1682–1771), professor of anatomy at Padua, conducted around 700 post-mortems in writing his *De Sedibus et Causis Morborum* (On the Sites and Causes of Disease) in order to show how disease was manifested within the organs of the body. His work was further developed by that of Marie Francois Xavier Bichat (1771–1802) in Paris, who as the 'father of histology'[3] located disease in the tissues, a step further on from Morgagni's emphasis on the organs. Bichat wrote in 1802 of the illumination available for the modern medic through morbid anatomy, over the traditional approach of the physician.

> For forty years from morning to night, you have taken notes at patients' bedsides on affections of the heart, the lungs, and the gastric viscera, and all is confusion for you in the symptoms which, refusing to yield up their meaning, offer you a succession of incoherent phenomena. Open up a few corpses, you will dissipate at once the darkness that observation alone could not dispel.[4]

Bichat's work shifted the centre of anatomical education to Paris. Toby Gelfand has analysed the new mode of anatomical instruction that grew out of the French schools, identifying the method as the 'Paris manner' of dissection.[5] This new approach allowed each student to undertake a dissection for himself rather than simply watching a demonstration. In Europe, and Paris in particular, there were corpses available for this personal dissection through the large public hospitals, where mortality rates were high and patients were assumed to have granted tacit consent on admission to hospital for post-mortem examination in the event of death. Additionally, and perhaps more significantly, private courses flourished in

Paris in the eighteenth century, and bodies were obtained through bodysnatching. One English student complained that due to the abundance, bodies were not dissected with care and attention: 'bodies are too plentiful and obtained at too low a rate, to be properly valued; and consequently most of them are rather *cut up* than dissected'.[6] Attempts to procure bodies at very low cost were successful largely due to the support of the French state for medical education, particularly anatomy, and to the early unification of the medical and surgical branches of the profession. This availability of corpses and the resultant exposure to anatomy led to large numbers of British medical men arriving in Paris for part of their medical education. The prominence given to dissection and the strong emphasis on the link with clinical medicine had a direct influence upon British medical students who made the journey, most notably Scottish medical men who returned home with an enthusiasm for pathological anatomy.

British Medical Education – Physicians

Eighteenth-century English physicians were the elite medical practitioners who established themselves in London, and occasionally in other cities, and charged high fees to the wealthy and discerning classes for advice, but never undertook surgical procedures or charged for prescribing medicines. The practice of 'physic' had traditionally involved itself with the internal condition of the individual, based on an imbalance between the 'solid fibres' and fluids of the body. Disease was usually ascribed to neglect of diet, constitution or exercise, and treatment was specific to each patient. Traditionally physicians rarely touched their patients beyond taking the pulse, and their claim to expertise was based on their ability to reason out the basis of disease and devise the appropriate treatment. Physic was not concerned with categorization or patterns of disease within populations, which became the province of surgeons and general practitioners.

For most of the eighteenth and nineteenth centuries the physician dominated the medical hierarchy in private practice as well as within the voluntary hospitals, but their position was ultimately in decline. In order to clarify the status of the two branches of medicine, it is worth noting that among practitioners with posts at major teaching hospitals, surgeons' pupils could not enter the medical wards, but physicians' pupils had the authority to visit surgical patients. Christopher Lawrence illuminated the dominance within this professional group of '*non-medical*' values: 'They worked in hospitals controlled by influential lay governors for whom research achievements were of relatively little importance. Men were appointed through nepotism or favouritism, as long as they were well-bred and soundly educated'.[7]

Physicians were socially privileged and held the most influential appointments yet were poorly educated in medical science. The emerging skills and disciplines of anatomy, physiology and pathology, based on observation and experience in clinical practice, were given less attention at the English universities during the era of reform than the long-established study of the ancient texts of Hippocrates, Aretaeus, Galen and Celsus. Traditionally physicians were gentlemen, and their education had been almost wholly literary, divorced from the manual labour of surgery. In 1834 the president of the Royal College of Physicians, Sir Henry Halford (1766–1844), commented on midwifery (practised often by surgeons) as an unsuitable activity for the physician:

> I think it is considered rather as a manual operation, and we should be very sorry to throw anything like a discredit upon the men who have been educated at the Universities, who had taken time to acquire the improvement of their minds in literary and scientific acquirements by mixing it up with this manual labour. I think it would rather disparage the highest grade of the profession.[8]

Paradoxically, during the seventeenth century, physicians had concerned themselves with post-mortem examination to establish the cause of death on their higher status private patients, particularly in London. Early examples are the scholar Isaac Casaubon in July 1614 and William Harvey in 1628 who undertook post-mortem work recorded in *De Motu Cordis*. Physicians, however, abandoned autopsies in the early eighteenth century, leaving the way clear for the growing band of surgeons to develop normal and forensic autopsy. It is tempting to speculate that the location of autopsy within the realm of the lower-status surgeon led to a hardening of attitudes to the opening of the body. The decline of English anatomy within the sphere of the physician meant that students wishing to develop their skills in dissection often had to undertake some of their education in Paris.

By the early nineteenth century English physicians usually received at least part of their training in Scotland, London or abroad. These centres began to re-introduce the importance of anatomy for physicians. Edinburgh University provided 'the most prestigious medical training, with its useful mixture of theoretical and practical instruction,'[9] which, unlike the English universities, conducted and examined in English rather than Latin, with no requirement for particular religious affiliation. Paris remained an important centre for anatomical instruction but was less popular for British medical students when there was an alternative. In the late eighteenth century Edinburgh University became the premier institution for the education of British doctors and held this position until the founding of the University of London. It was the first British centre to combine the educational benefits of a university medical school, private lecturers, its own royal colleges and large hospital facilities for clinical study. In 1800, of 600 medical matriculants at Scottish universities and Oxbridge, three-quarters had spent time training in Edinburgh.[10] The student attending the full medical course at Edinburgh University aspired to a gentlemanly ideal but was exposed to a surgical and anatomical approach that was absent at the English universities. This method developed out of the elevation of morbid anatomy within medical education, which rejected 'an earlier interpretation of diseases as general physiological imbalance' in favour of a 'clinical view of a specific disease linked to lesions observable at autopsy'.[11] The role of pathological anatomy and, therefore, dissection for physicians at the university and for surgical apprentices undertaking the same courses was strongly emphasized.

The 1792 *Guide for Gentlemen Studying Medicine at the University of Edinburgh* observed that anatomy was 'very properly considered to be the foundation of all medical studies', and Alexander Monro *secundus* (1733–1817), professor of anatomy, was attracting 88 per cent of Edinburgh medical students to his courses.[12] The prominence given to anatomy for all branches of medical study was certainly greater than that in England, but Edinburgh students suffered by comparison with Paris due to the difficulty of securing a supply of cadavers. Those autopsies that were conducted at Edinburgh were demonstrations undertaken by the professor or other academic staff. The anatomy lectures of Alexander Monro *primus* (1697–1767), professor at Edinburgh, were certainly popular and attracted large numbers, starting in 1726 with sixty-five and tripling that figure twenty years later.[13] This was achieved despite the use of just two cadavers each year. The poor supply was a catalyst to the development of private anatomy classes in Edinburgh in the early 1800s. This educational sector in Edinburgh was equally the province of the surgeon.

Surgeons

Surgeons and apothecaries had habitually been the inferior branches of medicine, concerning themselves with the external area of the body – notably cuts, wounds and fractures – and were viewed by elite physicians as tradesmen working with their hands. Many surgeons also treated venereal disease and acted as male midwives. The claims to greater respectability for the surgeon began with the severing of the union with the barbers in 1745 and elevation of their college to royal status in 1800. These moves largely benefited the small band of elite metropolitan surgeons who began to make claims for their great book-learning and liberal education, but a more general demand for better-educated and skilful surgeons and general practitioners came from the rank-and-file. Science took a man above mere trade, and elite surgeons often demanded the cultivation of 'moral attainments'. Joseph Henry Green, professor of anatomy to the Royal Academy and surgeon at St Thomas's Hospital, wrote that those aspiring to the medical profession should have the 'education, manner and habits of those with whom it should be his ambition to associate ... the gentry of the country'.[14] The key to success in surgery and general practice was seen to be a long training in anatomy and clinical medicine based on ward-walking, which distanced the expertly trained from the increasing number of unorthodox healers available in the crowded medical marketplace. The training of surgeons at the beginning of the nineteenth century reflected their lower status, with an array of opportunities centring on a compulsory five-year apprenticeship and a range of additional courses usually offered by private medical schools in London and the regions.

As an example, William Shippen of Philadelphia sent his son to the famed London surgeon John Hunter in 1758. Shippen Junior's diary illustrates clearly the commitment and hard work required as a medical apprentice in London: 'rose at six, operated till eight, breakfasted till nine, dissected till two, dined till three, dissected till five. Lecture till seven, operated till nine, sup'd till ten then bed'.[15] Clearly becoming a medical man was no easy matter, with years of hard work for the master surgeon, supplemented by private lectures and hospital attendance.

Richard Kay (1716–1751) provides more information through his own diary. His family background and training were quite typical of the eighteenth-century surgeon, with apprenticeship and a variety of voluntary courses. He was apprenticed to his father, a 'physician and surgeon' in Bury and Baldingstone, and his cousin was the first physician to the infirmary in Manchester. Richard spent a year at Guy's and St Thomas's hospitals in London and attended anatomy lectures and demonstrations.[16] Walking the wards in a large urban centre provided the opportunity to witness a variety of conditions while also providing access to bodies. These aspects of medical education became increasingly important for the successful surgeon and general practitioner at the ultimate cost of the apprenticeship.

The Royal Colleges of Physicians and Surgeons never showed an inclination to regulate training in any way, but the Worshipful Company of Apothecaries attempted some regulation of qualification by way of the licence to practise from 1815. This qualification, along with the diploma of the Royal College of Surgeons, was the aim of the surgeons and general practitioners. In order to prepare for such examinations, the candidates, in addition to the apprenticeship, chose from an array of opportunities in hospital practice and short private and hospital courses, leading to examinations for the apothecaries' licence (LSA) and the diploma of the Royal College of Surgeons (MRCS). By the first half of the nineteenth century, despite the poor legal regulation of medical qualifications, most surgeons had some sort of formal qualification with affiliation to a professional body, although there was no attempt by the royal colleges or the Apothecaries Company to monitor or inspect private courses.

Despite attempts to institute recognized qualifications, surgery's concern with manual operations and training through apprenticeship ensured that the connection with trade continued to affect claims to professional respectability. The position of even the elite surgeons at the beginning of the nineteenth century could be marginal next to the soundly educated physicians. One means for surgeons to aspire to the higher status of physicians was to claim a scientific supe-riority based upon anatomical knowledge gained through extensive dissection, thereby distancing themselves from the bulk of the surgical profession. Despite an alleged friendship with William Hey, surgeon of Leeds, Sir Astley Cooper declared that Hey was 'an ingenious man; but he had not that foundation in anatomy which fits a man for the highest scientific views of his profession'.[17]

Surgical Education – Private Anatomy Schools

The growing importance of qualification and certification as well as the rise in demand for skilled operators from the Georgian and Victorian middle classes offered a chance for ambitious surgeons to rise socially. This in turn provided the climate for private medical schools to thrive based on the example of France, where students were granted their own cadaver for dissection. Students in Eng-land during the late eighteenth century saw very few dissections and rarely got the chance to undertake an examination. Even in the prestigious Edinburgh University, one contemporary declared that there were very few bodies and those available were poorly preserved and exhibited:

> On the remains of a subject fished up from the bottom of a tub of spirits, are demon-strated those delicate nerves, which are to be avoided or divided in our operations; and these are demonstrated once at the distance of 100 feet.[18]

Another contemporary complained that 'there is always such a crowd of students about the physician and surgeon, that there is nothing to be seen or heard'.[19]

Private courses had been available for aspiring surgeons, usually in London, since the early eighteenth century, notably the classes of William Cheselden (1688–1752), who provided some means for hands-on dissection despite the difficulties imposed by the Company of Barber-Surgeons. He undertook eight dissections in London in 1717–18,[20] although the Company's by-laws prohib-ited dissection outside their own public exhibitions, and anatomists staging courses in their own premises risked prosecution until 1745. Those anatomy courses, where a lecturer anatomized 'a few dead human bodies and many animal bodies, living and dead', emphasized the study of natural philosophy and not the surgical method that grew out of the French influence.[21] The by-law prohibit-ing human dissection outside the Company of Barber-Surgeons lapsed when the surgeons set up their own College and thus assisted the growth of an increasingly competitive market in anatomical education.

William Hunter's education in Paris in the 1740s impressed upon him the need for medical students to undertake extensive dissection for themselves, and he was aware of the new opportunities for entrepreneurial teachers. He complained about the private and public dissections that allowed no personal experience, prevalent in London:

> I attended as diligently as the generality of students do, one of the most reputable courses of anatomy in Europe. There I learned a great deal by my ears, but almost nothing by my eyes; and therefore hardly anything to the purpose. The defect was that the professor was obliged to demonstrate all the parts of the body, except the bones, nerves and vessels, upon one dead body ... the operation of surgery was explained to very little purpose indeed, upon a dog.[22]

Hunter advertised his new anatomy course in September 1746 in the *London Evening Post*: 'gentlemen may have the opportunity of learning the Art of Dissection during the whole winter season in the same manner as at Paris'.[23] Thanks largely to Hunter, the Paris method of anatomy, whereby each student had a corpse to dissect for themselves, became the dominant form of private medical education in London. Ambitious medical men in the provinces, including Manchester, saw this method as a means to increase income and status and followed the trend established by Hunter.

Medical Reform in England and the Anatomy Debate

Although a 1540 Act authorized physicians to practise surgery, the acceptance of this tenet was much less certain in England even by the nineteenth century. In 1747 Robert Campbell claimed that physicians had to be able to supervise the work of inferiors.

> A young man, who has a mind to make a figure in the physical way, ought to learn, in some measure, all the inferior branches; that is, he must acquire a more than superficial knowledge in anatomy; not that it is necessary he should be entirely master of it.[24]

From this period there is evidence in England of an escalating call for science education, including anatomy, for the successful physician.

> To excel in it requires a greater compass of learning than is necessary in any other. A knowledge of mathematics, at least of the elementary part of them, of natural history and natural philosophy, are essentially connected with it: as well as the sciences of anatomy, botany and chemistry, which are indeed its very foundations.[25]

By the beginning of the nineteenth century the traditional divisions and competition between the branches of medicine were still much in evidence, but there were vociferous calls for a general reform in medical education, based upon the growing number of poorly educated doctors of all categories in a free market. Medical men, faced with a socially marginal position in society, published their views and within the debate often focused on the need for an increased role for anatomy. In an unregulated marketplace, many doctors saw anatomy as a means to claim expertise and elevate status. In 1759 Richard Davies expressed his concern over the 'most audacious quackery' practised in the name of medicine and the poor medical education available at Oxford.[26]

One of the earliest and most influential authors in the medical reform debate was the general practitioner Edward Harrison. In 1806 Harrison outlined the problem of physicians without proper degrees, surgeons and accoucheurs without 'proper instruction' and apothecaries without bone fide apprenticeships. He went on to complain that the medical profession would be 'relinquished ... to empirics and incompetent practitioners'.[27] His major concern was with what he saw as the increasing number of quacks and the decline in respectability of medicine as a career choice. This call for some type of regulation, and for stringent education and examination, led others to support his argument by outlining educational forms that elevated anatomy. Thomas Alcock, like Harrison, was anxious to 'increase the usefulness and respectability of the general practitioner' and greatly regretted the division of the branches of medicine. Alcock advocated extensive personal experience of dissection throughout the period of training, recommending nine hours of dissection each day for five days each week during a nine-month period of anatomical education. He said that 'pathological anatomy cannot be too highly valued as leading to improvement in the healing art', and he lamented the restriction of anatomy courses to the winter, which hurt poorer students who aimed to complete their training in as short a period as possible.[28]

Thomas Beddoes (1760–1808) wrote in response to Harrison's work and outlined a course of study that focused closely on the role of anatomy even for the physician: 'I propose to lay the foundation of medical education in the most exact mechanical and vital acquaintance with the human frame'. He claimed that all doctors had to be experts with the scalpel.[29] William Chamberlaine wrote that the medical student would have overcome any aversion to the dead body, as 'no person would undertake to repair a watch without being first acquainted with the structure of it'. Lectures alone were not enough, and the proper knowledge could not be achieved '*unless the pupil take the dissecting knife into his own hand*'.[30] Other authors were equally keen on the clock analogy and called for anatomical training for physicians: 'How incongruous and absurd would it be to suppose, that a man could discover an inaccuracy in the movements of a watch without knowing the proper arrangement of parts'.[31]

James Parkinson demanded of the medical student that 'anatomy ... must be your first and chief object'.[32] In an 1827 article on Guy's Hospital, the *London Medical Gazette* reported on the poor medical education available even in London compared to that available on the continent: 'The great deficiency in the education of medical students in England is in anatomical instruction'.[33] The writer claimed that students did not perform enough dissection themselves and lacked dexterity with the knife. Another influential article recognized that to survive in commercial society medical men had to offer genuine knowledge and skill in surgery in the face of inept and unqualified practitioners, and that physicians would have to embrace the new discipline:

> Anatomy alone will not teach a physician to think, much less to think justly; but it will give him the elements of thinking; it will furnish him with the means of correcting his errors; it will certainly save him from some delusions, and will afford to the public the best shield against his ignorance, which may be fatal, and against his presumption, which may be devastating.[34]

Thomas Southwood Smith (1788–1861) went on to assert that 'ignorant physicians and surgeons are the most deadly enemies of the community: the plague itself is not so destructive ... the basis of all medical and surgical knowledge is anatomy'.[35] This attitude was articulated most graphically by Sir Astley Cooper: 'he must mangle the living if he has not operated on the dead'.[36] Other influential doctors added their opinions, particularly during the 1820s when the debate over the Anatomy Bill was at its height. George Guthrie (1785–1856)[37] was adamant: 'It is agreed, that the study of anatomy, by professional persons, is indispensably necessary for the comfort and well being of mankind ... that the junior and inferior classes of medical practitioners should be at least tolerably conversant in anatomy'.[38] Certainly the *Medico-Chirurgical Review* recognized the trend: 'the number of works upon anatomy at present pouring from the press, argues an increasing taste or necessity for the study, despite ... the impediments and difficulties that now beset it'.[39] Thomas Turner, anatomy lecturer in Manchester, claimed that 'the study of anatomy and physiology is the key-stone to pathology and the healing art; and that without them, medicine and surgery would be mere empirical pretensions'.[40]

This new demand for anatomy was almost universally accepted, although even among surgeons (who were usually general practitioners) there was rarely a requirement to conduct a surgical operation. An article published in 1809 in a leading journal entitled 'Does a Minute Knowledge of Anatomy Contribute Greatly to the Discrimination and Cure of Diseases?' examined the move to elevate anatomy in the education of physicians:

> It seems to be the fashion ... to represent a knowledge of anatomy as the almost exclusive foundation of pathology and therapeutics; and to pretend to estimate the practical skill of the physician by the extent of his anatomical information.

The author directly disputed Beddoes's claim that anatomy was important for physicians:

> By far the major part of the science and art of medicine is altogether unconnected with anatomical information; and that the actual observation of the phenomena of

disease and the operation of remedies, is the great foundation of the physician's power and usefulness.[41]

The author of 'Observations on Medical Reform by a Member of the University of Oxford' demanded the preservation of the purity of physic and the medical hierarchy. He railed against the 'insolent tone of the medical reformers, as they styled themselves, by the clamorous audacity of their partisans, and by the levelling system they openly promulgated'.[42] The author feared that skill in anatomy could be a means of equalizing the status between medical practitioners, thereby diminishing the traditional respect given to the university-educated physician.

John Farre (1775–1862), founder of the London Ophthalmic Hospital in 1805, called for the study of morbid anatomy as there was too much emphasis on 'the anatomy of relative situation' in the schools.[43] Such attention could then be focused on hospital post-mortems demonstrating actual pathology and not just organization of parts. Even for surgeons, particularly beyond the very narrow group of elite practitioners, it was well understood that surgical operations were the last resort and to be avoided if at all possible. Surgery was, however, becoming fashionable, and one professional looked back with regret to his apprenticeship and ward-walking at St Thomas's in the 1820s:

> I have spoken chiefly of the *surgeons* of St Thomas's Hospital: and these were generally followed by the pupils, to the neglect of the practice of physicians and the study of medical cases, although it was of infinitely greater importance in its relation to the future and daily practice of their profession ... for every case of surgery, even of the minor order, that claims your attention, you will have forty cases of fever, and forty of other forms of bodily disease.[44]

The separation of anatomy from medicine was a minority view, and in the early nineteenth century Robert Graves (1796–1853)[45] lamented that 'the absurd idea that the education of a surgeon should differ from that of a physician [has] not been altogether abandoned'.[46] In the late 1820s the *London Medical Gazette* took up the cause of anatomy and championed the Anatomy Bill facing Parliament, fearing the dominance of Parisian instruction: 'The great deficiency in the education of medical students in England is in anatomical instruction'.[47] The 'prejudices of the public', ensuring the high cost of cadavers, hurt English anatomy when there was a perceived need for 'dexterity' with the knife.

The influential medical journal the *Lancet* was, from its inception in 1823, a strident supporter of the need for anatomy and dissection for medical students, despite the radical politics and opposition to the Anatomy Act of its founder and editor, Thomas Wakley (1795–1862).[48] In a lengthy article on the use of anatomy, normal and morbid, Wakley concluded:

In one word, it being admitted that the science of Anatomy is in a pre-eminent degree conducive to the happiness of mankind, and also that dissection of subjects is the best means of acquiring a knowledge of the science, it would be desirable to this end that subjects should be obtainable with the least possible difficulty.[49]

Much has been made of Wakley's hostility to the Anatomy Act due to its focus on pauper bodies, and this will be discussed in the following chapter; yet he was unwilling to abandon demands for better anatomical teaching.

Without that perfect knowledge of *the whole human frame*, of every vein and artery, muscle, nerve and bone – that anatomy only can give; the surgeon ... would find his efforts defeated, and valuable lives would be lost to society ... Such is the utility – the indispensable necessity, both to the physician and surgeon, of anatomy; a knowledge of which is only to be learned first, and then preserved by the frequent and continued dissection of dead bodies.[50]

The letters pages of the *Lancet* in the years prior to the Anatomy Act provide much evidence for the concern of doctors over their tainted association with the resurrection men and the desire for regulated anatomy teaching.

The elevation of anatomy in medical education in England was ultimately successful in the nineteenth century, resulting in the decline of the more experimental science of physiology. The fashion was for anatomy, but a more traditional role for the physician was not abandoned in Oxford before the end of the nineteenth century. Alongside the growing requirement for private anatomy instruction, there was a greater recognition of the role of the hospital in providing access to pathological anatomy through post-mortem examinations but more crucially in allowing contact with a large number of ill patients.

Hospital Medical Schools

In 1784 William Hunter (1718–83) predicted the future of medical success based on dissection and hospital practice:

Were I to guess at the probable future improvements in physic, I should say, that they would arise from a more general, and more accurate examination of diseases after death. And were I to place a man of proper talents on the most direct road for becoming truly *great* in his profession. I would choose a good, practical anatomist, and put him into a large hospital to attend the sick, and dissect the dead.[51]

In England, however, unlike Paris and other European centres, the development of the eighteenth-century voluntary hospital was a charitable movement focused on the benefits to the deserving poor. The philanthropist John Bellers observed in 1714 that three-quarters of the population were poor, and of the 200,000 who died each year, half were from 'curable diseases; for want of *Timely Advice*, and *Suitable Medicines* ... It's as much the Duty of the *Poor* to Labour when they are Able, as it is for the *Rich* to Help them when they are sick'.[52] During the later nineteenth century, medical men gradually increased their influence and were permitted to admit increasing numbers of clinically interesting cases, but the beginning of the hospital movement was characterized by lay managers and governors and concentrated services on those deserving poor who were likely to recover. Consultants in English hospitals were honorary appointments, unlike their European counterparts who were full-time and salaried and therefore able to devote time to teaching and research. As a result the aim of improving medical knowledge was a recognized but minor focus until later in the period, and there was little opportunity for dissection and post-mortem examination.

Bellers wrote that hospital deaths would educate the doctors: 'when anyone Dies in the *Hospital*, their Bodies should be opened, for the better information of the *physicians*';[53] but medical education was not a primary aim of English hospitals. A published letter from Thomas Percival (1740–1804)[54] reflected on deaths in hospitals: while one-third of the Paris population died in its hospitals (one-fifth in the Hotel Dieu), the figures for St Thomas's and St Bartholemew's were one in thirteen, Northampton one in nineteen, and Manchester one in twenty-two.[55] In 1819 John Abernethy, surgeon at St Bartholemew's, told a meeting at the Royal College of Surgeons:

> The indigent who suffer from illness and injury are supported and relieved chiefly by the liberality of that benevolence which is so creditable to our national character, and as much as I wish for the promotion of medical knowledge, I should be sorry if the bodies of the poor were to be considered as public property ... in our country. Far better would it seem to me, that medical science should cease, and our bodily sufferings continue.[56]

Edinburgh University did manage to follow a more European model of clinical instruction described by Hunter, with the hospital at the centre of education and research, complemented by a range of lectures and demonstrations offered at the medical school which correlated closely with clinical observation.[57] The promotion of this approach was usually dependent on a great number of cadavers available, as in Paris with its high hospital mortality rates, although the private schools of Paris were still partly dependent on bodysnatching as in England and Scotland. Edinburgh managed to some extent to overcome its lack of cadavers due to innovative teaching methods. Useful clinical teaching was also dependent on the growing power of medical men in hospitals to control admissions and management of patients. The London hospitals were able to offer ward-walking opportunities, and between 1725 and 1815 over 11,000 pupils applied to the London hospitals for access to the wards.[58] It is difficult to gauge the level of access to cadavers for dissection, although the more limited post-mortem operation that had greater public acceptance at these larger hospitals may have proved a reasonable source of anatomical training, backed up by private courses supplied by bodysnatching. The role of hospital teaching will be examined later in this chapter and in Chapters 4 and 5, but it is apparent that Oxford University failed to develop a strong relationship with the Radcliffe Infirmary. There is, however, evidence that anatomy was initially a recognized academic discipline at the university.

Oxford Anatomy

Physicians at Oxford and Cambridge underwent long and expensive training based on a classical arts education; at Oxford in 1833, seven years were required for graduation in the Bachelor of Medicine degree and another three for Doctor of Medicine. This qualification gave Oxford and Cambridge graduates a particular benefit over graduates of Scottish and European universities, through their unique ability to become fellows of the Royal College of Physicians of London. Two-thirds of those graduating Bachelor of Medicine from Oxford in the first quarter of the nineteenth century became fellows of the Royal College. Michael Durey has termed the Oxford medical education 'antidiluvian' because 'undue emphasis was still placed on the value of a literary education and a respect for ancient authority'.[59] As a result the two English universities were eclipsed by the rise of medical education in Paris and Edinburgh, with their high regard for the study of anatomy and their provision of a student's personal experience of dissection for both physician and surgeon.

As early as 1549 there was a recognition that physicians at the University of Oxford needed to undertake dissection. The statutes drawn up after Edward VI's visitation in that year demanded that each medical student had to view two dissections and perform two more before he could practise. For a Doctor of Medicine degree, a student had to undertake a further three dissections. There was no requirement that these should take place in Oxford of course, but in the seventeenth century Oxford was something of a centre for scientific study, and growing interest in the human body allowed a minor flourishing of anatomy. This was not the result of efforts by the university but of interested private teachers. Private instruction in anatomy at Oxford grew out of the anatomical enquiries of notable scientists Thomas Willis (1621–75), Christopher Wren (1632–1723), Richard Lower (1631–91) and Robert Boyle (1627–91). Willis wrote *Cerebri Anatome* (1664), illustrated by Wren (dependent on extensive human dissection), and Boyle first preserved human specimens in alcohol. Lower carried out the first blood transfusion after making dissections of the heart (*Tractatus de Corde*, 1669) and conducted a lengthy correspondence with Boyle after the latter's removal to London. The letters describe many animal anatomies and illustrate the anatomists' willingness to undertake dissection on whatever materials might be available whenever bodies were scarce. In 1664 many sheep were dissected after an epidemic disease made them cheap, and Lower was given an 'interesting' kidney from a butcher's shop.[60]

Prior to the Anatomy Act all social classes were in danger from bodysnatching, but the true threat fell largely on the poor. This area will be explored in Chapter 3, but the little evidence which exists for early human dissection in Oxford suggests that these noted anatomists were able to utilize a higher class of body drawn from private patients. Lower wrote to Boyle about the 'ventricles of the brain', with drawings done by Wren, on a case of Willis's when 'the whole body was opened'.[61] Further dissections were conducted on a fellow of a college, a scholar's head, a gentleman of All Souls College and Lady Littleton's son.[62]

Later in the period the necessity for dissection was often disregarded by elite physicians of Oxford. Certainly the Regius Professors of Medicine had abandoned the tradition of performing regular anatomies long before 1690, and up until 1800 the professorship was regarded as little more than a sinecure, with incumbents undertaking private practice in distant locations and leaving the requirement to lecture on Hippocrates or Galen twice a week to an assistant. In common with Edinburgh and London, private courses in anatomy were available from the seventeenth century, given by Lower, Willis and their followers, such as Christopher Furneaux (d. 1729), William Musgrave (1655–1721), Edward Hannes (d. 1710), James Keill (1673–1719) and James Monro (1680–1752), as well as visitors from Switzerland, Scotland and London. One Oxford personality, Frank Nicholls (1699–1778), began lecturing in Oxford between 1719 and 1721 and managed to secure the Tomlins Readership in Anatomy, earning the title, praelector in anatomy. Yet the rewards of private lecturing in London were too great a draw for Nicholls, and he left for the metropolis in 1727. William Hunter attended Nicholls's lectures in London in 1740 but was unimpressed at the use of only two bodies in thirty-nine lectures. Nathan Alcock (1707–79) attempted to re-establish anatomy teaching at Oxford in the face of declining support from the university establishment.

These efforts at private teaching in Oxford were limited, and given the few bodies available, they were likely to have involved animal dissection to a great degree. In 1710 Conrad von Uffenbach visited Oxford and attended a dissection by D. Lavater (son of the professor of medicine at Zurich). He reported that the anatomist had to resort to lecturing on osteology as he 'had no corpses to dissect (which he was hoping to obtain from London)'.[63] By the time Matthew Lee died in 1755, leaving an endowment for the foundation of the Lee's Readership in Human Anatomy and a new anatomy building, the university as a centre for the study of science and medicine was in decline, and there was no greater commitment to dedicated medical education. Despite the 1636 Royal Charter allowing the university the body of any person executed within twenty-one miles around

Oxford, the supply of cadavers was always a problem: after becoming Lee's Reader in Anatomy, John Kidd (1775–1851)[64] 'procured permission to lecture from models and preparations'.[65] The supply of dissection material at Oxford is examined more closely in Chapter 2.

The first Lees's Reader in Anatomy, Dr John Parsons, was appointed in 1767. As a physician, he delegated his first dissection to John Grosvenor, anatomical surgeon, but provided the accompanying lecture. His opening address illustrates the 'high style' of anatomical studies at Oxford.

> That when considered with respect not only to the professions of surgery and medicine, Anatomy is of use to men of other professions has been advanced and such a position may very well be supported ... To all men whose professions require the aid of eloquence and oratory it must be of use in common with other studies for furnishing that copiousness of language which the knowledge of many sciences will abundantly supply, and that brilliancy and vivid colouring which in oratory is to be produced by a judicious assemblage of proper and chaste metaphors collected together with accuracy from every branch of science.[66]

This lengthy quotation demonstrates that lectures on anatomy, under the terms of the Lee will and despite the decision to build a dedicated anatomy school, were no more likely to address the development of morbid anatomy at Oxford. Such lectures were to be valuable to the natural philosophers of Oxford, illustrating the glory and greatness of God, and were not seen as particularly beneficial for the growing demands of dissection-centred medical study. Anatomy and dissection lectures were regularly attended by students aspiring to the clergy. The only existing Oxford student diary containing sparse references to anatomical lectures from the seventeenth and eighteenth centuries was written by Bryan Twynne, who became the vicar of Rye.[67]

The age and traditions of the University of Oxford made it difficult for anatomy to find favour in medical study. In 1835 Adolph Muehry observed the classical nature of study in Oxford:

> When one sees Oxford with its two and forty colleges, large, antique structures; where the gardens with their evergreen shrubs, bushes and banks, the broad courts strewed with yellow sand ... when one sees all the circumstances inviting to retirement and study ... the libraries so well fitted for abstraction and forgetfulness; the painted windows of the chambers where the student may waste the midnight oil and watch the return of day ... one cannot but wish that other objects of science might here fill and employ the heads, which are content now in busy idleness, to pore over the classics of Greece and Rome.[68]

Professor John Kidd was much criticized in contemporary accounts for the lack of anatomical focus in Oxford medical education. Dr C. G. Carus, physician to the King of Saxony, visited Oxford Anatomy School in 1844, by which time the school was moribund; he described Kidd as lecturing to one university student and the odd apprentice from the town in anatomy from wax models and bought preparations.

> Professor Kidd, a good-natured old gentleman ... he may, probably, formerly, have had some talents, or at least some liking for personal activity and inquiry; at a later period, without any excitement from without, in a University devoted almost entirely to philology and theology (which is, indeed, no *universitas*) and without the sufficient inward power and excitement, the stagnation of all philosophical study of natural history soon put a stop to his activity.[69]

When Carus talked of the latest techniques in anatomy in Europe, Kidd 'complained bitterly that so little interest for these subjects was exhibited in Oxford, and gave hopes of renewed activity'.[70] Kidd informed the University Commissioners in 1848 that students had been going to London for the theory and practice of medicine for forty years.[71] Yet it seemed that Kidd 'could not make any way against the predominating classical stream'.[72] The traditional ideals of Oxford were appropriate when there was a demand for learned and literary physicians, but they were of little use when the discipline of anatomy and the pursuit of empirical study became fashionable.

Oxford University accepted that it would not be a major centre for clinical teaching and saw its role increasingly as providing preliminary preparation for more specialized training in London. Clinical Professor James Ogle (1792–1857)[73] admitted that 'the wider range and more ample accommodation of the London schools' were more suited to professional studies.[74] Kidd informed the Select Committee on Medical Education in 1834 that 'there was no necessity in the University to require attendance on all those forms and lectures in Oxford, which had become of no value when its students had resorted to better schools of medicine'.[75] It was, however, a good platform for making useful contacts. In 1806 the mother of a prospective Oxford medical student was advised that:

> His medical education will not be improved by this plan, for there are no lectures of reputation upon any branch of medicine given at Oxford, however, he will ... become acquainted with the manners and the people of this country, may form some connections which may be of use to him in future life, and will more easily advance his profession when settled in London.[76]

Henry Wentworth Acland (1815–1900),[77] who went on to become a luminary of Oxford medical education in later life, was advised by Sir Benjamin Brodie (1783–1862)[78] to attend Christ Church, Oxford, for his first degree and then go on to St George's in London for his clinical training.[79] In Acland's case, money was no object to this expensive course of study. The later offer of an academic career at Oxford was received with concern by his father, Thomas Acland, who wanted a more glittering career for his son based on his status as an elite physician:

An extensive and lucrative practice in London, with possibly an appointment at the Court, the fame derived from scientific researches, the applause of crowded audiences at one or another of the great medical schools – these were objects worthy of a young man's ambition. But to settle down at the age of forty as a teacher of science in a place where science commanded scant respect – with the chance of a limited practice in the town and surrounding neighbourhood – may well have seemed an inadequate fulfilment of early aspirations.[80]

William Hunter developed a highly lucrative career as an anatomist and accoucheur and so never achieved the high status derived from fellowship of the Royal College of Physicians. Despite his success, he wished for higher social rewards for his own relatives: he sent his younger brother to St Mary's Hall, Oxford, in 1755 and his nephew, Matthew Baillie, to Balliol College.

Oxford University as a whole went into a severe decline in medical student numbers from around 1670, with the 470 enrolments of that year falling to below 200 a century later.[81] Oxford students still had to subscribe to the thirty-nine Articles of the Church of England until 1856, which ensured that only Anglican candidates presented themselves at the university for the major part of the nineteenth century. Most importantly for medicine, however, was that the university was dominated by a classically based education designed for clerics and lacked the will to reform this situation in line with developments in medical education in Europe and Scotland. Oxford medical students had to obtain an arts degree prior to any medical studies, and the Bachelor of Medicine was rarely achieved in less than eight years. In a letter to the *Lancet*, 'a retired general practitioner' praised this situation:

It is the glorious beauty of an English university that, before any man can obtain its degree, in any science, he must have passed through that course of general education and acquired that knowledge of literature, both ancient and modern, which constitutes *the well informed gentleman*.[82]

Prebendary Gaisford (1779–1855), dean of Christ Church College (1831–55) (home of the Anatomy School), outlined the advantages of the classical education: 'It enables us to look down with contempt on those who have not shared its advantages, and also fits us for places of emolument not only in this world but the next'.[83] There was much pride in the length of time it took to obtain a medical degree at Oxford, when a similar qualification could be achieved in three or four years at Edinburgh. The author of an article in the *Pamphleteer* caused much outrage with his comment that 'a Scotch physician so easily gets the degree of doctor and a Scotch surgeon is so much upon this level, that his next aim is to be on a level of the English physician'.[84] Much of this article and this particular quotation illustrated the author's concern with the increasing merging of physic and surgery.

Such attitudes isolated Oxford University until late in the century and injured its medical education, particularly after the foundation of the University of London, which won the right to confer medical degrees in 1836. Robert Masters Kerrison, along with many other contemporary authors, championed the opportunities available in the metropolitan centres and condemned the education at the English universities where there was 'no *efficient* school of medicine or anatomy in either University'.[85] The *Lancet* supported this position: 'it is far from my wish to detract from the merits of our English Universities; but will anyone pretend that medical knowledge of any utility is to be obtained there?'[86] Other centres were able to provide better opportunities by exploiting the relationship with local voluntary hospitals that could provide access to clinical medicine. Oxford University was unable to capitalize on the initial educational hopes of the founders of the Radcliffe Infirmary.

Hospital Education in Oxford

In 1770 the Radcliffe Infirmary was established, and the university did make an attempt to follow the European and Edinburgh model by appointing the first holder of the Lichfield Chair of Clinical Medicine in 1780. The professor was expected to attend the wards of the Radcliffe Infirmary and examine the patients alongside a set of students and provide clinical notes. In 1839 the Chairman of the Committee of Revision of the Rules looked back to the initial aims of the founders, where there had been a recognition that education was to have a particularly strong presence at the infirmary:

> This Infirmary was originally intended for educational as well as charitable purposes, and ... it is honourably distinguished from most other provincial infirmaries of that early date (with respect to the end contemplated by those who contributed to such institutions) by the fact that professional instruction was from the very beginning one of the objects embraced by the foresight of the good and able men who forwarded and effected the erection of the Radcliffe Infirmary ... it cannot be said, as it has been said of others, viz 'that professional education is an excrescence on a charitable institution' (*London Medical Gazette*, vol 17, p 25) ... the Radcliffe Trustees having built their Infirmary 'for the improvement of the art of medicine'.[87]

The voluntary hospitals of the university towns were at first seen as a means to improve poor medical teaching. One year after the opening of the Radcliffe Infirmary, Cambridge was endowed with Addenbrooke's Hospital, and in the opening sermon the clergyman (later the Bishop of Gloucester) commented 'that charitable hospitals might deflect contemporary criticisms against English Universities, where only theoretical medical instruction was given, obliging many young men to seek training outside England'.[88] Yet the medical school within the Radcliffe Infirmary went into a severe decline from the middle of the nineteenth century, despite its supposedly strong beginning. This will be examined further in Chapter 5. In Manchester there were encouraging opportunities for clinical education at the infirmary, but the town's initial success in medical education was based firmly on independent anatomy schools with a ready supply of cadavers.

Manchester Anatomy Schools

The growth of Manchester as an influential urban centre in the later eighteenth century was reflected in the proliferation of medical institutions often initiated by medical men. By 1834, in addition to the infirmary established in 1752, Manchester boasted a children's hospital, the Ardwick and Ancoats Dispensary, the Salford and Pendleton Dispensary, the Lock Hospital, the Eye Hospital, the Manchester and Salford Lying-In Charity for delivering poor married women in their own homes, and the Manchester Medical Society. Medical education in Manchester was focused on private anatomy schools (which grew out of the Literary and Philosophical Society) as an adjunct to apprenticeship, providing practical skills for students who might find opportunities for walking the wards in Manchester (at the infirmary from the 1790s), but who would generally go on to further study in a major metropolitan centre. Charles White gave some of the first anatomy lectures and demonstrations in 1783 at the College of Arts and Sciences in Manchester.[89] Medical students, particularly in the regions, were the trainee surgeon-apothecaries or general practitioners who lacked the prestige of the physician. The medical schools of Manchester were therefore solely concerned with the education of surgeons and surgeon-apothecaries (general practitioners) through apprenticeship and private courses.

Among the pioneers of provincial medical education was Joseph Jordan, born in 1787 into a family of calico printers in Manchester and apprenticed to an infirmary surgeon at the age of fifteen. He received the diplomas of the two Edinburgh medical colleges and joined the First Battalion of the Royal Lancashire Regiment. By 1811 he was studying in London but returned to Manchester in the following year to become a junior partner in a medical practice. This lasted just two years, and in 1814 an advert appeared in *Wheeler's Chronicle*: 'to students of anatomy, Mr Jordan will open rooms for the study of anatomy on the first of October. Bridge Street'.[90] Competition did not arrive until 1824 with the establishment of Thomas Turner's school in Pine Street, and Jordan had to expand his curriculum, but his focus was always anatomy. Yet Jordan was only able to continue this private school until 1836, when Turner took over both schools to form the Royal Manchester School of Medicine and Surgery.

Thomas Turner was born in 1793, the son of a banker in Truro. He was apprenticed to Nehemia Duke, a surgeon in Bristol, and later became a student at Guy's and St Thomas's under Sir Astley Cooper, then studied in Paris, attending the great hospitals for the winter and spring season 1816–17.[91] Turner arrived in Manchester in 1817, having chosen the city because his sister had settled there. He was appointed as house surgeon to the Lunatic Hospital and Infirmary, responsible for seventy-four medical and surgical patients along with a further twenty out-patients and twenty to thirty house patients each day. Four years later he gave up this post and established his own practice as well as giving lectures at the Literary and Philosophical Society on anatomy, physiology and pathology. Permission was granted by the Society, but 'no dissections be allowed'.[92]

It is interesting to note from the foregoing few facts the different experiences of the two men. Jordan, from a relatively humble background and training despite his local connections, found it difficult to establish himself in clinical practice in Manchester and turned to teaching to establish a career. Turner, on the other hand, experienced a more exalted level of surgical education in London and Paris and was able to establish himself in Manchester with little difficulty, and his clinical practice came before his establishment in education. Turner and Jordan are good examples of the entrepreneurial medical man, exemplified by William Hunter. Both men turned to teaching as a means to social advancement and lucrative honorary hospital appointments in a city that, after 1815, became medically overcrowded. Pertinently, Thackray has characterized Manchester at this time as a city of 'social isolation, political emasculation and tumultuous surroundings'.[93] Manchester was turbulent, far from the metropolis and without political representation until the Reform Act of 1832. The teachers' adoption of the role of anatomical lecturers was one means of distancing themselves from the distinctly marginal position of the bulk of provincial surgeons.

Jordan's stated aim was to save students and their families the cost of courses in London, and he also successfully appealed to the fear of moral laxity in the metropolis. It was generally felt at this time that 'amusement is necessary to young men. If this be not enjoyed at home and within themselves, they will fly abroad into company and seek it, in taverns, in conviviality, and dissipations'.[94] The *Manchester Guardian* echoed these sentiments, calling on parents to be aware of 'the moral danger of placing the charge, unwatched, amidst the seductions and temptations of the metropolis' and advocating local medical education.[95] Jordan's course was approved by the Apothecaries Society in 1817 and by the College of Surgeons in 1821, as 'One special advantage was claimed by Jordan for his school: bodies or subjects for dissection could be obtained very easily'.[96] Willis Elwood and Felicite Tuxford have claimed that Jordan was so successful in obtaining cadavers that he sent surplus bodies to Knox, the doctor later implicated in the Burke and Hare case.[97] Their work is poorly referenced and much of the evidence is at best anecdotal, but it is certain that bodies were discovered on stagecoaches bound for Edinburgh, and these claims will be explored further in the next chapter.

Thomas Turner was one teacher who advocated the elevation of anatomy for surgical students, but he was also keen to ape the higher learning of the physicians, with their fluency in Latin and Greek as well as mathematics and natural philosophy, in addition to chemistry, botany, anatomy and physiology:

> Our profession has its *real* dignity, and the power to command respect; but it has no claim to those qualities unless the members of it have such acquirements, as will enable them to perform all the duties of their important calling.[98]

Like Jordan, Turner wished to elevate teaching in Manchester and save students from the need to attend schools in London:

> It is hoped that the necessity of a departure to such a distance from home will soon cease to be necessary, and that the pupils of Lancashire and the adjoining counties, will have the means of improvement very near at hand.[99]

Turner believed that students needed opportunities for conducting their own dissections and echoed many of the proponents of educational reform:

> For it is by dissection only that the student can gain that minute acquaintance with parts which is necessary for practical purposes. It is only by researches leisurely conducted, and by the use of his own knife, that he can determine where he may use the scalpel in the living body with freedom, and without fear of dangerous consequences, and when to cut would be to kill his patient.[100]

Although Stephen Anning has claimed that the 'first complete medical school in the provinces ... was that opened in Manchester by Thomas Turner in 1824, which became in 1836 the Manchester Royal School of Medicine',[101] both Jordan and Turner were aware that their schools were 'preparatory' ones and students would have to go on to study at the 'superior' schools of London and Edinburgh. After the 1815 Apothecaries Act, the Society of Apothecaries generally encouraged provincial schools and recognized Manchester as the premier of its ilk: John Watson, secretary of the Society of Apothecaries, reported to the 1828 Select Committee on Anatomy:

> No young men came before the Court of the Society of Apothecaries better qualified in every respect than those who had been entirely educated in Manchester, where excellent lectures on every branch of medicine are given by competent teachers and the Manchester Infirmary affords, under the physicians belonging to it, most ample opportunities for the acquirement of practical knowledge.[102]

Numbers were small; between 1830 and 1833 Pine Street School only had twenty-three candidates for the Apothecaries exams compared to St Bartholomew's 249, although Butler has pointed out that the provincial schools played 'a significant role in educating the local profession. Over half the practitioners educated between 1810 and 1860, who later joined the honorary staff of the Manchester Infirmary attended one of the local schools'.[103]

The College of Surgeons proved to be a harder nut to crack after 1815, when it increasingly protected the status of the London surgical elite. In 1822 the Royal College refused to recognize dissection taking place in the summer, arguing that the practice was a health hazard to students and the wider public. This was a direct attack upon the private schools, where anatomy was taught throughout the year to reduce costs. Student numbers were dropping in London as students left for Paris and greater access to bodies, and so the hospital teachers of London moved against their competitors in the provinces, namely the private schools that had provided popular practical training. In 1826 the College of Surgeons in London failed to recognize Thomas Turner's courses. Presenting themselves as the upholders of scientific standards, the reply from the college illustrates a determination to protect the metropolitan hospital teachers from encroachment by outsiders:

> This Court regret that they cannot allow his certificates to be so admitted, because if they allow it to him they must allow the same to every person who shall lecture in any provincial town, which, in the opinion of this Court, would be detrimental to scientific professional education.[104]

Generally the college would acknowledge lectures held at the universities of Dublin, Edinburgh, Glasgow and Aberdeen or at the recognized London hospitals. Turner was indefatigable in his efforts, however, and in 1829 the Edinburgh College of Surgeons recognized his year's course in anatomy, midwifery and 'attendance upon the hospital', and the London College followed suit in 1830 for anatomy and physiology. Nevertheless, the provincial schools operated under a great disadvantage due to college by-laws which allowed for reduced study and clinical periods in London.

The staff of the Manchester schools and the Manchester Royal Infirmary clearly felt that the institutions in the city were a special case and should have been dealt with by the Royal College of Surgeons differently to the other provincial schools. A further consideration by the Royal College was that hospital attendance had to be at one of the recognized schools with an attached hospital with 100 beds. The college would recognize certificates of attendance on provincial hospitals with 100 beds, but only if the student had previously attended two courses of anatomy lectures and two courses of dissection in a recognized school of anatomy. The hospital attendance had to be twice as long for provincial (as opposed to metropolitan) hospitals. The *London Medical Gazette* acknowledged the anomaly, as many provincial hospitals had double the number of beds of a recognized centre like Aberdeen.[105] Thomas Wakley pointed out the absurdity of qualifying as a surgeon with twelve months at the Westminster Hospital with only eighty beds, as opposed to the four years it could take to qualify in a provincial town with a larger hospital. He also noted that all four surgeons at the Westminster Hospital were on the Council of the Royal College of Surgeons.[106] Turner wrote again in 1830, and on this occasion his courses in anatomy and physiology were recognized. Joseph Jordan's courses on anatomy, physiology and surgery were accepted in 1831.

The struggle over the infirmary was protracted. On 21 October 1830 the infirmary formed a committee of Dr Bardsley, Mr Wilson and Mr Turner to request that the Royal College of Surgeons recognize the certificates of attendance on the hospital. The letter of 21 October 1830 requested that 'the Institution ... may henceforth be placed on the same footing with respect to the Certificates of Attendance on its practice, as the recognized hospitals in London, Dublin, Edinburgh, Glasgow and Aberdeen'. In support of their application, the doctors who signed the letter cited royal patronage, a greater number of patients than any other provincial institution, the age of the institution and its size, with 180 beds, 100 fever beds and eighty lunatic beds. The infirmary also laid claim to scientific superiority: 'that from its acknowledged reputation in the advancement of science, and the advantages derived from the great number of patients, this Infirmary has now become an extensive School for Pupils in Medicine and Surgery'.[107] The Royal College's Court of Examiners considered the application and replied:

> It is very gratifying to the Council to witness the zeal and anxiety evinced by the medical officers of the Manchester as well as of many other Provincial Hospitals and Schools to promote the views of this College, in advancing the education of their students and consequently the eventual good of the public; they will always be ready to continue their encouragement of these schools of which they have already endeavoured to give the strongest proofs, and which have hitherto been duly appreciated but they do not under present circumstances feel that they are justified in exempting the Hospital and School of Manchester from the general regulations adopted with respect to Provincial Hospitals.[108]

The reply was disappointing, and the committee resolved to try again. Royal patronage was once again emphasized and had been obtained as a result of the 'wealth, population and scientific character of the town'. It was claimed that students had the benefit of a 'greater number of surgical opportunities ... than in any other hospital in the kingdom', and that the infirmary contained more beds than some of the 'privileged hospitals'. The letter emphasized the expense of a London medical education and finished with a warning:

> Should our present application unfortunately prove as fruitless as the former one, it will be evident to you, that as we consider our claim to be founded in justice, no other resource will be left to us than to represent our case to the Legislature of the Country.[109]

A final verdict from the officers of the college was not received until March 1831: 'With every respect for the Officers and Teachers of Manchester, they do not feel themselves justified in exempting their Hospital from the operation of those Rules'.[110] The Manchester Committee felt aggrieved enough to address a petition to the House of Commons. The complaint was one of unfair treatment by the Royal College, with its recognition of twelve months' hospital attendance in London, Dublin, Edinburgh, Glasgow or Aberdeen, or alternatively six months in one of the above plus six months in a provincial hospital.[111] The anomaly was not reversed until 1845 when the Senate of the University of London was authorized by the Home Office to accept hospital practice certificates from the Manchester Royal Infirmary.[112]

Hospital Education in Manchester

Manchester Infirmary was founded with fifty beds, and like all other voluntary hospitals, it was a charitable institution for the deserving poor. Admittance was gained by the recommendation of subscribers to the charity and not by medical need or interest. There is little evidence in the minutes that the doctors were able to use the patients as clinical research material, and post-mortem anatomizing was not acceptable to the management committee. Thomas Fawdington (1795–1843),[113] when physician's clerk to the infirmary, was reprimanded in 1818 by the Weekly Board of Governors for opening up a patient's body without permission; the Board was 'highly disappointed of his conduct in this and other matters'.[114]

There was a growing struggle between the honorary medical staff and the lay trustees during the early 1800s. The government of the infirmary remained under the dominance of its lay treasurer, J. L. Phillips, who 'regarded the Infirmary surgeons and physicians as self-interested' and felt that the lay trustees were the key to serving the best interests of the infirmary.[115] There is little evidence in the minutes of the infirmary from the early 1800s to suggest that there was any particular interest in medical education. Apprentices of the local surgeons were able to walk the wards with their masters, but there were no formal clinical lectures at the infirmary in the early half of the century. The medical education that developed focused on anatomy and was firmly in the hands of individual medical entrepreneurs.

Conclusion

This chapter has afforded an opportunity to explore the extent and expansion of medical education by the beginning of the nineteenth century, prior to the passing and implementation of the 1832 Anatomy Act. It provides some explanation for the introduction of legislation, without some of the source problems experienced in other chapters more dependent on primary material. It opened with a discussion of the development of medical education in Europe and illustrated the spread of anatomically focused instruction. It has, in particular, aimed to offer a picture of the education available to English doctors at two extremes of the educational spectrum, in the local context – an aspect that has, until recently, been missing from the published record. Within that focus, it has questioned the supremacy achieved by anatomy in the medical curriculum by examining the eighteenth-century debate over minute anatomy. Finally, this chapter has examined the rise of the hospital medical school, where anatomy could be efficiently taught with ready access to clinical cases and cadavers. These developments took place well before the passing of the Anatomy Act.

This work outlines the initial dominance of Oxford in the education of physicians when physic was at the top of the English medical hierarchy. By examining medical education in Europe, this chapter illustrates the changing nature of education for physicians and the growing need for anatomical proficiency. These developments were to hurt the University of Oxford, with its emphasis on physic and its refusal to adapt to changing circumstances. Had the university actually possessed the will to adapt, however, it would have been unable to procure the necessary materials to establish a significant anatomy school. The following chapter examines Oxford's access to dissection material prior to 1832 to illustrate this point. Manchester concerned itself with the education of surgeons based on anatomical expertise, and as such was following a new fashion in medical education. The city saw the foundation of provincial medical education due largely to the efforts of ambitious medical men who saw education as a way to increase income and status in an overcrowded profession. They used their position as teachers and their roles within the new Royal Infirmary to demand recognition from the regulatory bodies on a par with that given to schools and hospitals in the established centres. In order to establish successful anatomy schools, however, access to dissection material was vital, and it is this supply which is examined in Chapter 2.

It would appear that Oxford University failed to foresee the nineteenth-century transformation of medical education and remained a limited, provincial medical school for physicians who would have to complete the bulk of their training elsewhere. The development of clinical medicine in such a small town was inevitably limited, as the body supply would always be difficult and the naturally strong link with the Radcliffe Infirmary was never exploited. The provision of clinical material for teaching was theoretically possible through the infirmary, but voluntary hospitals, managed as they were by lay governors, saw their responsibility as protectors of the deserving poor, and not primarily as offering centres for clinical instruction. The Radcliffe Infirmary at Oxford, more than most, was dominated by clergymen who took that role particularly seriously and even after the passing of the Anatomy Act forbade dissection of bodies. The key medical men of Oxford within the university and the infirmary were, moreover, steeped in the tradition of the learned and gentlemanly practitioner. Although some of them presented themselves as men of science, it was a limited interest in the study of natural philosophy and not a claim for increasing the role of laboratory medicine.

Despite the huge changes taking place in medical education in Europe, with the rise of pathological anatomy and the attendant laboratory sciences, Oxford – and to a lesser extent Cambridge – remained content during the nineteenth century to continue their traditional roles. They were essentially concerned to allow young men to make excellent social contacts and to prepare them for undertaking a particular social and professional standing in metropolitan society.

The Manchester schools should have benefited from the new trend in anatomical expertise and surgical competence. The schools were hurt, however, by the metropolitan bias of the Royal College of Surgeons, which only recognized the London anatomical schools of their senior members. The Manchester teachers did eventually succeed in having their courses recognized, but the city remained a centre for preliminary training prior to study in London, Edinburgh or mainland Europe, until the adoption of medicine into Owens College in the 1870s.

2 DISSECTION IN OXFORD AND MANCHESTER: SUPPLY AND DEMAND BEFORE 1832

Having seen the growing importance of morbid anatomy to the education of doctors in nineteenth-century England and the responses to this in Manchester and Oxford, we can now examine whether the basic material was available to students and what effect supply had on medical school development in the early part of the period. This chapter will examine two themes: firstly, the legal and illegal supply of bodies in Manchester and Oxford (allied with the growing dominance of anatomy within the medical curriculum); and secondly, public attitudes to dissection.

Despite the problems in revealing covert body supply, it has been possible to uncover a rough approximation of legal supply of bodies to surgeons despite the difficulty of using the assize records. This has been done through an examination of the local press in Oxford and Manchester, as trials were covered in detail by *Jackson's Oxford Journal* and the *Manchester Guardian*. For Oxford, Thomas Hearne's contemporary account[1] is extremely illuminating, detailing trials that resulted in hangings and ultimately in anatomization, as well as describing instances of bodysnatching in the city. The clandestine nature of bodysnatching results in very little obvious evidence of the practice, unless the state was successful in prosecuting resurrection men. Again the local press is extremely useful in documenting successful and unsuccessful bodysnatching incidents. A reading of parish records for Oxford also illustrates that local churches were concerned with the sanctity of burial grounds. The records of the Manchester Medical Collection indicate that some medical men built up large anatomical collections that were almost certainly partly the result of undocumented instances of bodysnatching (as well as more obvious post-mortem operations).

Despite the expansion of dissection, there was no legal means of obtaining large numbers of cadavers prior to 1832. Hanged criminals of all categories were available (but difficult to secure) until 1752, when the Murder Act confined the source to murderers and gave anatomists the right to claim them. The aim of this legislation was largely punitive, and it did nothing to increase the supply of bodies at a time when the medical profession was growing. The very few people sentenced to hang for the crime of murder in England could not possibly satisfy the increasing demand.[2] Up until this date there was no automatic right to bodies from the gallows. Between 1805 and 1820, 1,150 people were executed throughout Britain, yet there were over 1,000 medical students in London alone.[3] This disparity left anatomists to grapple with members of the crowd who would often attempt to rescue the hanged criminals. There was huge competition at the gallows between the Royal College of Physicians, the Barber-Surgeons Company and the private anatomy schools in London, all vying for a body with family and friends who would also try to claim it. These struggles were apparent in Oxford during the eighteenth century and are examined in this chapter, illustrating the difficulty the local medical men experienced in procuring bodies for anatomization.

The need for a greater number of bodies ensured that grave robbery became the main source of dissection material, and the organization of the resurrection trade reached its highest level in London, with professional gangs working in competition from the late eighteenth century to provide for the private schools of anatomy. Historians of London bodysnatching can draw on first-hand accounts, including a surviving diary by a bodysnatcher and evidence given as part of the Select Committee on Anatomy.[4] Other centres have been somewhat neglected, partly because the evidence is less abundant, and this study of Manchester and Oxford is limited by the inevitable reliance on reports of failed attempts at bodysnatching reported in the local press and trial proceedings. As we will see, however, the different role of dissection in the curriculum in the two places probably had a substantial impact on sources of body supply, with Oxford remaining content to produce the increasingly rare pure physician, and Manchester mirroring the experience in London and other urban centres with the rise in the role of surgery. Oxford was able to depend on a small supply from the gallows for part of the period but certainly had recourse to bodysnatching, and its difficulties here ensured that even its limited needs were not met. The Manchester schools had little supply from the hangman and depended more directly on the trade in bodies, emerging as a major centre for bodysnatching activities, with resurrectionists able to supply local surgeons as well as participate in the transportation of bodies to other centres. My research would indicate a national trade in bodies, a contention articulated by Elizabeth Hurren in her work on Cambridge University and by MacDonald in her book examining the Anatomy Act at work in Scotland, England and Australia.[5] An examination of hospital minutes allows an insight to the supply of bodies available from this source, one which was highlighted by Richardson and further demonstrated by MacDonald.[6]

The elevation of the mastery of the disciplines of anatomy and surgery within the development of the medical profession was concomitant with changing attitudes to the treatment, and specifically burial, of the poor. Pauper funerals became starker ceremonies as the wealthier classes sought to limit expenditure on the poor rates, allowing for the eventual arrival of the Poor Law Amendment Act. The loss of the right to burial in the local churchyard and the tightening of access to ceremonial aspects of the funeral for the poor was another assault upon those people most at risk of bodysnatching and dissection. Funerals displayed less ostentation during the nineteenth century, but the inviolability of the grave and the observance of traditional funerary custom remained important to individual and family respectability. Again, although Manchester, with its large industrial population, experienced the effects of this more immediately, the poor also felt and voiced their vulnerability in Oxford.

Bodies were difficult to get hold of, and there are contemporary accounts of the problems common to English anatomists:

> The aversion of the English to anatomical dissections is another of the prejudices which characterize that nation. The surgeons have great difficulty in procuring dead bodies: they are obliged to pay large sums for them, and are forced to carry them to their houses with utmost secrecy. If the people hear of it, they assemble in crowds around the house, and break the windows.[7]

In both Manchester and Oxford it is possible to discern the attitude of the population and the difficult relationship existing with the medical fraternity. The population of Oxford apparently remained largely acquiescent even during the cholera epidemic and the passing of the Anatomy Act, while that of Manchester resorted to a major riot when emotions were heightened due to the outbreak of the disease. The next chapter examines the well-known riot against the medical profession in Manchester at the time of the cholera outbreak in 1832 and the passing of the Anatomy Act. The present chapter investigates the implications of the rioting against the enclosure at Otmoor by Oxford people during the early part of the nineteenth century. Both illuminate the concerns of the poor over the perceived changing attitudes of the wealthier classes as well as specifically over murder and dissection.

Legal Supply of Cadavers and the 1752 Murder Act – Oxford

By the eighteenth century there were around 160 crimes punishable by hanging, which gave the medical men a large pool of possible dissection material. They, of course, had no particular exclusive right to a body until 1752, although the law of the land allowed them to make a claim to each body. As is illustrated in this chapter, bodies were fought over by relatives and friends anxious to spare the hanged prisoner from the final humiliation of dissection even after the passing of the Murder Act.

There are two early and interesting cases from Oxford that resulted in a possible benefit for the condemned. In 1650 Ann Green, a maidservant, was hanged in the Castle Yard at Oxford for smothering her illegitimate child.[8] Green's body was taken to the Anatomy School at Christ Church for dissection, where the reader in anatomy, William Petty (1623–87), and his associate, Thomas Willis (1621–75), managed to revive her, and she lived into old age.[9] This must have been something of a disappointment to Dr Petty, who rarely received a body for dissection. According to Hearne, he usually 'cut up dogges'.[10] John Aubrey remembered that Dr Petty 'kept a body that he brought from Reading a good while to read on, some way preserved or pickled'.[11] Green's revival took place despite a hanging of a quarter of an hour, and 'while she was hanging, divers friends of hers and standers by, some hung with their whole weight upon her, others gave her great stroakes on the breasts; and moreover a souldier did the same severall tymes with the butt end of his musquett'.[12] Her story inspired a popular verse among the university students:

> Ann Green was a slippery queen
> In vain did the jury detect her; –
> She cheated Jack Ketch, and then the vile wretch
> 'Scap'd the knife of the learned dissector.[13]

It was later concluded that Green was innocent, and her baby was probably stillborn. Ten years later another maid was hanged for the same crime in Oxford, and she was sent to Dr Conyers for dissection. He revived her, but she was not as fortunate as she was seized by the bailiffs and hanged again successfully.[14]

Green's case illustrates the conflict that took place at the gallows between anatomists and supporters of the condemned. Most hanged criminals were anxious to avoid dissection. Vincent Davis pleaded with the mob to save his body: 'I have killed the best wife in the world, and am certain of being hanged, but for God's sake, don't let me be anatomized'.[15] In 1719 the only person hanged at the Oxford Assizes was a man of twenty-two from Thame. His parents brought a coffin but were beaten by the scholars, who 'took the body by force, abused the Father and Mother in such a degree that the woman miscarried'.[16] The body was dissected by Christopher Furneaux (d. 1729) at Exeter College (adjacent to the anatomy school in the Ashmolean Museum). In 1730 Richard Fuller was hanged at Oxford for murdering his wife. Medical students demanded the body, but it was given over to the felon's friends and 'a desperate riot ensued', with the students seizing the body. It was recovered by the proctors and sent in a boat to Caversham, where it was once again seized and taken to Christ Church. There the body was 'made a skeleton and the flesh dispersed up and down'.[17] Although hangings were rarer than in the metropolis, violent scenes between anatomists and the crowd were apparent in Oxford before 1752.

The aim of the 1752 Murder Act was to increase the severity of the punishment for killings over other crimes, and as such the guilty would be anatomized or hung in chains. In 1759 at Surgeons Hall, Mr Tate, surgeon, read over the body of Richard Lamb, who had been executed for murder. The purpose of the Act was not to increase the supply of subjects but 'to strike a greater terror into the minds of men, not by inhuman tortures on the living subject, as in other countries, but by denying the murderer the privilege of having his bones rest peaceable in the ground'. Tate also referred to the rarity of the crime of murder, even in London, and said over the body of Lamb: 'this is but the second subject executed for murder, committed in this large and populous city and county, for upwards of two years'.[18]

After the Murder Act Oxford seems to have been a little more successful than Manchester in claiming bodies, probably due to its status as an ancient university permitted to undertake public dissections by claiming 'a sounde body of one of the executed persons'.[19] The Act helped the claims of physicians to bodies from the scaffold but did not stop public protest. Even after the Murder Act there are examples of anatomists attempting to claim the bodies of hanged murderers without success. In 1754 the bodies of the highwaymen Bryce and Briscoe were rescued by friends and relatives despite the attentions of the anatomists.[20] The execution of the highwayman Isaac Darkin (also known as Dumas, 'Prince of Highwaymen') in 1761 resulted in another defeat for the anatomists. *Jackson's Oxford Journal* reported the rescue of the body by the Oxford bargemen:

> His body was carried off in triumph by the bargemen and most inhumanly mangled in order to prevent (according to his own request) his being anatomized. Could he have foreseen this treatment, he would perhaps have shown less reluctance to become the subject of *nicer operations*.[21]

Darkin had apparently 'declared that he feared – not death – but the thought of being anatomized'.[22] These cases illustrate not only the rarity of bodies from the gallows for the Oxford anatomists but also the strength of feeling within the population against anatomization. The crowd, while accepting the execution of the criminal, would not stand by and allow the anatomists easy access to the corpse.

A survey of the Calendar of Prisoners at the Oxford Record Office revealed just six dissected criminals between 1788 and 1832, including Edward Thorn of Henley, executed on 28 July 1800 for poisoning Amey Jacob, 'his servant, (who was far gone with child by him)'. A broadsheet reported:

> After hanging for the usual time his body was cut down, and immediately conveyed to the Anatomy School to be dissected and anatomized, according to the law of the land, with respect to persons convicted of the foul crime of murder.[23]

Regrettably for the anatomists, murderers were rare in rural Oxfordshire.

A legal supply of bodies from the gallows may, however, have been one factor in the decision to establish the Oxford Anatomy School at Christ Church College in 1765. Matthew Lee's will provided the capital for the establishment of the Lee's Anatomy Readership.[24] Under the terms of the will, the reader had to be a Westminster student at Christ Church and a layman studying medicine at Oxford, and resident in the town for at least half the year. The duties included teaching two courses of anatomy each year. The will stated that the reader 'shall dissect at least one adult human body and distinctly explain and regularly demonstrate all the bones, viscera, blood vessels, muscles, nerves and all other parts of the human body with their respective uses'.[25] Dr Lee also provided the sum of forty pounds towards the expenses of making anatomical preparations and procuring bodies.

The Christ Church Anatomy School did manage to build up a museum of anatomical specimens, and the Christ Church archives demonstrate this. A 1794 letter identifies sections of kidney at the school, and in 1806 an entry notes two preparations, 'one of the head and nerves of the face, the other of the thorax and abdomen laid open to shew the visceral nerves etc ... placed in the Anatomy School in or about 1806'.[26] In 1800 'the head of an old woman' was purchased for one pound and four shillings.[27] There are several other instances of items placed in the school, but there is little evidence of the promised whole-body dissections demanded by the Lee will, although the salary of twenty pounds for courses in dissection was paid regularly and it should be noted that the records are scanty prior to 1832. The evidence from the Anatomy School records is of an increasingly difficult supply of bodies at the beginning of the nineteenth century.[28]

Legal Supply of Bodies – Manchester

The anatomists in Manchester had great difficulty in claiming bodies from the gallows. In 1826 Elizabeth Bate was murdered at Winton, near Manchester, by Alexander and Michael McKeand of Manchester, who were convicted at Lancaster on 21 August. The local newspaper reported, 'we believe several applications from individual surgeons were made to the sheriff for the bodies, but he declined granting any of them. He ordered one to be given up to the surgeons at Lancaster'.[29] The body of William Robinson, hanged in Lancaster, was given up to the surgeons in 1827,[30] and that of Jane Scott from Preston the following year.[31] These examples again demonstrate the rarity of consigning condemned criminals to the anatomists after the Murder Act and the fact that some cases benefited the surgeons at the Lancaster Infirmary and not the anatomists in Manchester.[32]

The Manchester surgeons do not seem to have had any sort of supply from the gallows until 1831, when Moses Ferneley, executed at Lancaster for the murder of his stepson in Manchester, was sent to the infirmary at Manchester for dissection.[33] After a body was designated for dissection, it was usually sent to the surgeons at a hospital. It would seem that the private anatomy schools, the main source of anatomy education in Manchester, did not have sufficient official authority to claim bodies from this source, although the key personnel at the hospital were of course the owners of the Anatomy School and may have invited their private students to attend at the hospital or passed on the body after dissection at the infirmary. There is very little evidence that the anatomists in Manchester received a reasonable supply of bodies through legal means. There were certainly few available for newly established private anatomy schools. It would therefore seem likely that the need for bodies in the private schools led to the development of a flourishing trade in cadavers, and this is examined later in the chapter.

Bodysnatching in Oxford

The late eighteenth century saw the rise of the private anatomy school, with men like William Hunter (1718–83)[34] providing demonstrations on the 'Paris model', whereby each student dissected a body for themselves rather than simply observing the master at work. The growing demand for hands-on dissection encouraged teachers to look towards an unlimited supply in the local churchyard. Bodysnatching was probably started by individual medical students who provided their teachers and themselves with subjects. Joseph Jordan, founder of private medical education in Manchester, certainly claimed that 'the students in my time were obliged to steal bodies'.[35]

Bodysnatching tarnished the reputation of the medical student in the public eye. One contemporary account from the United States claimed that 'the public considered every medical student as a potential bodysnatcher, and put them in a social class that was taboo', which led to students attempting 'to try to live up to this reputation'.[36] Punishment for those stealing bodies, particularly medical men and students, was lenient, as the body itself did not represent goods or possessions, and sentences were light. The first indictment for bodysnatching in 1777 in London caused confusion over the law. After much wrangling between defence and prosecution over the category of the crime, felony or misdemeanour, the judge, Sir John Hawkins, agreed that there was no property involved and sentenced the defendants to six months' imprisonment and whipping, calling it a crime 'contra bonos mores' (against decency and good manners).[37] Professional resurrection men were careful not to remove clothing or grave goods, which could result in a much harsher sentence.

Previous studies have suggested that London alone was a major centre for bodysnatching. Lisa Rosner contended that 'cadavers were hard to obtain in Edinburgh'.[38] A contemporary student wrote in 1810, 'in Monro's class, unless there be a fortunate succession of bloody murders, not three subjects are dissected in the year'.[39] Christopher Lawrence has noted that Monro *primus* developed innovative teaching techniques to alleviate the problem of cadaver supply:

> For several years the Professor of Anatomy had many difficulties to struggle with such as 1. Penury of subjects for his course. 2. A general prejudice of the people to dissections of human bodies, who foolishly believed that he stole living people to dissect them alive.[40]

Monro *secundus* complained that students at other institutions 'had the benefit of dissection'.[41] Anatomists would, however, always complain of shortages. Lawrence believed that the situation in Edinburgh was alleviated as the century wore on, and MacDonald supported this contention, arguing convincingly that the anatomists in Edinburgh made more extensive use of infirmary bodies.

In Oxford, unlike Manchester, instances of bodysnatching are difficult to find. Hearne (1678–1735), antiquarian, sub-librarian of the Bodleian and keeper of the Anatomy School, provides some evidence for the eighteenth century. Around 1710 a woman was disinterred from St Peter's Churchyard in the East by students:

> being some way or other disturbed as they were going along, they dropped her and set her in her shrewd, bolt upright, just under Edmund Hall against the wall, where (before day) in the morning she, being seen frighted some people, who knew nothing about the matter.[42]

He also noted a dissection of a snatched female body on 14 May 1715 performed by a visitor from London.[43]

There is evidence that several parishes were concerned with the possibility of bodysnatching in Oxford. The St Martin Carfax vestry minutes record the election of a watchman at the church in 1798, to be paid by public subscription and to be provided with a lantern and rattle.[44] In 1808 All Saints followed this example by appointing Thomas Hine.[45] However, the bulk of the evidence suggests that the supply of bodies prior to the Anatomy Act was very difficult for Oxford, despite the confidence engendered by the building of the Anatomy School. John Bellers in his famed treatise wrote: 'At present its not easie for the students to get a Body to Dissect at Oxford, the mob are so Mutinous to prevent their having one'.[46] This is further illustrated by a foreign visitor to the early Anatomy School in the Ashmolean Museum. Zacharias Conrad von Uffenbach wrote of a 1710 visit to the Schola Anatomica to see animal specimens:

> When a dissection takes place (which, as is universal *in publicis lectionibus*, scarcely ever happens) it is never here but, as the *custos* himself stated, in one of the other schools, possibly so as to prevent the collections here from being injured or even stolen.[47]

Thomas Hearne, the *custos* in question, had been much annoyed the previous year by the vice-chancellor's decision a year earlier to allow a visitor, Dr Sandilands (or Sandolans or Sandelands) from Scotland, to undertake dissection in the Anatomy School when several treasures had been stolen. Unusually, Hearne noted that Dr Sandilands ('a good anatomist')[48] had several bodies to work upon, and this abundance was something of a nuisance over the six-week visit:

> Great offence was given last year to strangers that came to the Library, who could not endure the smell that was caus'd by the Bodies being cut up; that this Year there was like by such operations to be greater offence by reason of the Rifeness of the small Pox, tho' indeed last Year the Persons concern'd were so inhumane as to let the Bodies of children lye so long in the school that the worms bred in them.[49]

Sandilands obviously had no difficulty in procuring a reasonable supply of bodies, including most interestingly those of children, which were particularly prized due to their rarity. It is tempting to speculate that these bodies may have come from London, given the relatively short distance involved, but unfortunately nothing further is known about Dr Sandilands.

Hearne also stated that the resurrection of the body disinterred at St Peter's in the East, Goody Beecham,[50] was a mistake as the snatchers had wanted a much younger woman who had been buried at the same time. He noted that the bodies of young women were a particular target, and there was obviously some concern over this in Oxford in the early 1700s. A few years earlier the wife of the college cook had been buried within the church:

> The reason of her being buried in the Church was to prevent her being taken up again, it being a common practise nowadays for young physicians to rob church yards, tho' even churches are still less safe, many Clerks, as 'tis said, in London, and other great places, being confederate with the physicians.

In 1999 archaeologists discovered a pit behind the original Ashmolean Museum (the present Oxford Museum for the History of Science) where official Oxford University anatomy lectures and demonstrations took place during the seventeenth and eighteenth centuries. The pit contained material cleared out before the move to the newly built Anatomy School at Christ Church in 1767. The excavation uncovered over 2,000 human bones (representing no less than fifteen individuals) as well as 600 bones from at least twenty-three individual dogs, a figure considered to be very high by the archaeologists.[51] This collection has remained a mystery to the excavators: 'the group remains ... enigmatic but on balance is probably associated with laboratory activities'.[52] Bill White, human bone specialist and member of the archaeological team, suggested that the condition of the human bones and the presence of children's bones implied that the bodies may have come from bodysnatchers rather than the gallows, but this conclusion is no more than an opinion.[53]

On permanent display in the Oxford Museum for the History of Science is a skull from the dig that is of particular interest. The trepanned skull demonstrated further growth after the operation, proving that that the patient survived at least a few months. This would indicate both a close relationship between the clinician caring for the patient and the anatomist, and a tracing of the patient through to death, allowing for ultimate dissection. Again this would suggest that the body was snatched rather than being that of a convict.[54] There is also evidence that a small pit existed for the disposal of remains at Christ Church in the early 1800s. A visitor to Sir Christopher Pegge (1765–1822), Regius Professor of Medicine from 1801, was 'permitted to examine the receptacle in which the bodies are deposited after he has finished lecturing on them ... and to remove all offensive smell a little stream is turned through it'.[55] Dumping bodies behind the anatomy school at Oxford was obviously the norm, suggesting that public fears over the lack of final burial for dissected bodies were entirely justified.

In the early nineteenth century there is little evidence for resurrection activities within the city of Oxford, but several cases do appear in the local press from the environs. The only case found in this study of a conviction for bodysnatching in Oxfordshire surviving in the Oxfordshire Quarter Sessions records is of a resurrection gang operating in Caversham in 1830. The Quarter Sessions rolls for Lent 1830 note that William Davis, William Bedgood and Richard Knapp, all labourers, were convicted at the assizes of taking the body of William Matthews on 20 November 1829. Bedgood and Knapp were found guilty of a misdemeanour and sentenced to twelve months' hard labour in the house of correction.[56] There is no direct evidence that such events were intended to benefit the anatomists at Christ Church, but there are reports of local incidents close to the town. In 1830 bodysnatchers were disturbed in Banbury:

> An attempt was made on Friday night last to carry away a body from Banbury churchyard, which was fortunately prevented by the vigilance of the watchman. A reward of ten pounds has been offered for the apprehension of the offenders by the Churchwardens.[57]

On 19 November 1831 the Oxford paper reported on a body found in the possession of resurrectionists. It was that of Eliza Bates, aged eleven of Wingrave near Aylesbury, who was later reinterred.[58]

The anatomists at Oxford obviously attempted to find bodies wherever possible, but the numbers involved even in the archaeological findings are small. The rector of Lincoln College complained in 1810:

> As to the *clinical lectures in medicine*, liberally endowed by a late Chancellor of the University, though the Reader is a Physician of the first practice in Oxford, and of

undoubted skill, he has not been able to raise a single class for the last two or three years; though that class should only consist of the number six.[59]

By 1834 the Regius Professor of Medicine, John Kidd, was complaining of the lack of cadavers, which made adhering to the terms of the Lee bequest of dissecting two bodies per session very difficult. His evidence to the Select Committee on Medical Education claimed that no dissection had taken place for five or six years as 'it has been impossible to get a subject'.[60]

Bodysnatching in Manchester

Manchester anatomists, by contrast, seemed to have little problem in finding cadavers: Joseph Jordan advertised openly in the *Manchester Guardian* for students for courses of lectures on anatomy and physiology, 'dissections as usual'.[61] G. A. G. Mitchell, in an article reminiscing over his student days, claimed that the Manchester anatomy teacher Joseph Jordan supplied Dr Knox in Edinburgh and was once fined twenty pounds and besieged in his anatomy school for 'instigating bodysnatching', while the resurrectionist involved received one year's imprisonment.[62] In an article for an academic journal, Jordan wrote of his regret at being unable to give full details of the case being discussed, as 'we could not obtain much information on the symptoms which attended this unusual state of the circulation; the body having been raised for the purpose of dissection, we were precluded from seeking for information from his relatives'.[63] Jordan's nephew, who was his apprentice and later partner, stated that 'the supply of subjects was always abundant, even greater than required'.[64] The other notable Manchester anatomist, Thomas Turner, made similar claims, obviously in an effort to elevate his own anatomy school:

> The means of dissection which our school affords gives to it a superiority over the schools of London and Edinburgh. We have never wanted the means; they have. My pupils have dissected until they grew tired of it; and the London and Edinburgh pupils have grown tired and disgusted from the want of it. It must be so when young men go to London and crowd those places, entirely ignorant of anatomy, for the supply is not adequate to the want.[65]

Turner published several illustrated books and papers on anatomy (in addition to a book and article on medical education) demonstrating the use of dissection material.[66] Thomas Fawdington, founder of the Marsden Street School in Manchester in 1829, published an illustrated book detailing a post-mortem discussed later, as well as an extensive catalogue from the anatomy museum at the school.[67] Within the catalogue there are hundreds of items listed from cadavers of all ages, including foetal material. Many items must have been received from bodysnatchers, although two aortas were received from Dr Carbutt at the infirmary; and there were obviously donations from other doctors, for example a six-month human foetus that came from Dr Frederick Hutton of Staley Bridge.[68] Some may have been received directly from patients, including a 'human ovum about the fourth month'.[69] The anatomists also had access to organs and body parts from post-mortem operations conducted at the Manchester Infirmary. The large museum collection, valued at two thousand pounds, was bought by the Manchester Infirmary on Fawdington's death.[70]

The Manchester Medical Collection contains an undated catalogue from Joseph Jordan's anatomy museum in Mount Street listing around one thousand items. Like Fawdington's catalogue there is much foetal material, and some items that must have been received from bodysnatchers, including 'the scull of a man who was brought into the dissecting room in the year 1824. Individual unknown' and 'the calvarium of a child who was brought into the dissecting room in 1828 ... the child appeared to have died of bronchitis'.[71] One skull had been removed from a grave after seven years, as the grave was re-opened to inter the occupant's brother.[72] Again, there are items brought in from other medical men and body parts of Jordan's own private patients and organs taken from hospital post-mortems.[73] Jordan's catalogue is of particular interest due to the size of the collection and the notes on sources, many of which indicate snatched bodies.

Bodysnatching in Manchester started as an activity conducted by individual medical men and their apprentices. In 1825 the *Manchester Guardian* reported on the discovery of a suspicious character lurking around Hulme burial ground on the edge of the city and who was apprehended by the deputy constable. The man 'turned out to be a young man of respectable family, and an apprentice to a surgeon in this town'. He was discovered with several unexplained tools 'apparently for the purpose of disinterring bodies'.[74] In these cases punishment was often lenient but became harsher once the trade was professionalized. One celebrated case in Manchester was that of John Eaton, sexton of St George's chapel, the subject of a broadsheet and publication, who was convicted in 1827 for the felony crime of stealing a child's coffin. He received six months' hard labour.[75] William Penkethman, convicted of stealing a dead body from Alderley Churchyard in Cheshire, was not so fortunate in 1831. He received a sentence of two years' imprisonment in Chester Castle.[76]

The newspaper evidence points to Manchester being an important centre of bodysnatching activity often for onward transport to other areas.[77] The *Manchester Guardian* reported in 1824 on the trial of two men discovered packing boxes with bodies for transport to London. The difficulty of securing a prosecution is illustrated by the comments of one lawyer, who 'observed that he thought the stealing of bodies was undoubtedly a misdemeanour, yet the finding of them in a man's possession was not sufficient to warrant his commitment, unless they were proved to be stolen'.[78] These six bodies were bound for London, as was a body discovered in 1826 at the Pickfords Manchester warehouse.[79] On one occasion two dead bodies were discovered aboard the Lancaster coach en route to Edinburgh. They were in a box loaded at Manchester, and discovery only took place due to the 'very offensive smell which proceeded from it, and several passengers complained'.[80] Manchester also received bodies: in 1825 the *Lord Blaney* steam packet arrived from Dublin containing a trunk with the bodies of a woman and child inside.[81]

By 1830 the trade in bodies was becoming controlled by working-class gangs who could see the obvious financial rewards to be gained. The infamous Burke and Hare received around ten pounds in winter and eight pounds in summer for each of the bodies murdered for Dr Knox in Edinburgh in 1828.[82] One doctor recorded the activities of Manchester students with some understanding, but had no sympathy for the bodysnatchers: the students' 'macabre activities still evoke feelings of repulsion, but their ends were laudable ... no such excuses can be made for the professional resurrectionists who scraped a precarious livelihood from one of the foulest trades in human history'.[83]

In 1830 James William Home was committed to the New Bailey prison in Manchester for stealing a body from Bolton; 'from papers found in his possession, it appears that he has been for some time in the regular practice of supplying Dr Knox, the well known Edinburgh lecturer on anatomy, with subjects from this neighbourhood'.[84] In 1831 a body was discovered in a Manchester warehouse secured in box bound by iron hoops and directed to 'Mr John Smith, Edinburgh, to be left till called for'.[85] Of those cases of bodysnatching that were discovered and therefore received coverage in the press, the great majority were destined for onward transportation to other locations, and they were probably uncovered due to the difficulty of arranging parcelling and transportation. The risks were obviously worth taking, and bodysnatchers became increasingly audacious. The *Manchester Guardian* reported on the theft of the body of 'Old Tom', a well-known street character. The unfortunate Tom had frozen to death on Deansgate, a principal thoroughfare, while begging and selling matches. His body was then stolen from a nearby house by three men claiming to be relatives. Not only had the bodysnatchers posed as kin, they had also taken an incredibly distinctive body, as Tom was well known as a veteran of the Greenland whale industry and had wooden legs. The body was never found, indicating that anatomists did not ask too many questions about the origin of the bodies they were lucky enough to receive.[86]

In 1832, John Doherty (1798–1854), editor of the radical Manchester paper *The Poor Man's Advocate*, conducted a campaign against one Mr Gilpin, rector of nearby Stockport, accusing him of supplying his brother-in-law, a surgeon, with bodies.[87] The threats of a libel case did not dampen Doherty's determination to expose clerical connivance:

> Jesus and G-lp-n, so 'tis said
> Both in their turn have rais'd the dead,
> The former broke the chains of death,
> The latter rais'd them without breath,
> One gave them back to light and life,
> The other to the surgeon's knife.[88]

The bodysnatching incident that provided the first spur for parliamentary action in 1828 took place in nearby Warrington, Lancashire. This is examined in more detail in the following chapter.

Bodysnatching was a vital source for Manchester anatomists, but public anxiety and the resulting high costs of bodies meant that there were periodic shortages. At these times the teachers could utilize their own museums, which have been discussed earlier. The museum catalogues illustrate the wealth of material available within Manchester's anatomical museums, collected by industrious anatomists over years of practice and available to their many students over numerous years. These formed an important collection that could aid claims of provincial institutions to be at the forefront of anatomical knowledge, and although used in conjunction with the autopsy, they could be studied independent of the vagaries of supply. It seems likely of course that the contents came out of surgical operations and full-body dissections, and Jonathan Reinarz claims convincingly that 'many interesting specimens could be harvested from the least fortunate members of the English population, the sick poor'.[89] The evidence from Manchester certainly supports his work on Birmingham. Of course one other source, already noted for Manchester, may have been from bodies available through hospitals.

Hospital Bodies

It has been suggested that the new voluntary hospitals provided an important resource for the anatomists, and therefore much of this section will deal with the contextual literature on this subject. There is certainly much anecdotal evidence to support the contention that hospitals could provide a useful supply of bodies. One medical student at Bristol in the 1820s claimed that:

> As many acute and fatal cases were admitted, and there was an autopsy in nearly every case of death, there were abundant opportunities of getting a practical knowledge of all the viscera, and also admitting of dissections of many parts without any apparent injury or disfigurement of the body.[90]

The student, Alford, enjoyed regaling his readership with the japes of his youth. There was no dedicated medical school in Bristol at the time, but a course of anatomy lectures was held in a private house some way from the hospital, from where corpses were stolen: 'We supplied a sufficient number of subjects for dissection from the Infirmary dead-house, by removing the bodies from the coffins and putting in some substitute'. The London Hospital was apparently also 'notorious' for raiding its own mortuary.[91]

What cannot be known with any certainty is the use made of the post-mortem examination in hospitals as an aid to the teaching of anatomy. MacDonald's recent work on Edinburgh illustrates that the Royal Infirmary was a vital resource for Edinburgh anatomy schools.[92] The Bristol medical student Alford wrote with enthusiasm about the use of the autopsy when full dissections were not possible, and there may not have been the same level of concern within the population over the idea of a limited post-mortem examination to discover cause of death; indeed it could be used as a tool by the coroner to investigate medical men and hospitals. Russell Maulitz believed that there was a difference in the public mind:

> There was a clear distinction between the practice of obtaining bodies for conducting teaching dissections and the practice of conducting the examination ... while the former was abhorrent to a sizable part of English society (an echo of the special fate awaiting the remains of hanged murderers) the latter was tolerated at least in principle.[93]

Post-mortem examinations were certainly accepted by the public when they were used to establish cause of death in murder investigations.[94] John Farre advocated the more extensive use of the routine post-mortem examination, stating rather optimistically that:

> All persons, who have had opportunities of judging the fact, are aware, that little or no opposition is made to the post-mortem investigation of disease, by the friends of the deceased. All private and personal feelings are sacrificed to a noble sense of the public good.[95]

Ian Burney has written convincingly, however, that even the coronial autopsy was unpopular and numbers were low.[96] John Mann's *Recollections* illustrates the attitudes of Irish patients under the care of the St Thomas's Hospital physician John Elliotson in the 1820s. The Irish population had a particular objection to post-mortem examinations and often removed the bodies of relatives from the hospital immediately after death, as 'they feared that a portion would be retained'.[97] This fear was justified, as Mann noted a home post-mortem examination on an Irish patient where the brain was removed, hidden in a handkerchief, and placed in the St Thomas's anatomy museum.[98]

MacDonald's research on Edinburgh and London anatomy supports the contention that hospitals and asylums always provided much post-mortem material. She notes that relatives were less likely to object to an operation that was considered to be limited in scope and dedicated to finding a cause of death. The clinicians, however, often had wider aims and would, in any case, often act without direct permission.[99] The autopsy is used today as a teaching tool, and it is tempting to suggest that it was ever thus.[100] McDonald's research, however, relates to a later period when the Anatomy Act was creating cadaver shortages for private schools, and privileged anatomists turned to their own hospitals for supplies of post-mortem material and teaching.

The public image of the late eighteenth-century hospital was imperative to its survival, dependent as it was on voluntary contributions from the community. There may have been an early belief, as Richardson states, that 'to many, to enter hospital was synonymous with death' and ultimately dissection.[101] In her study, fear may have been deeper and more prolonged among the poor, as her focus is on London. Richardson's contention that these institutions were the key to supplies of cadavers before and after the Anatomy Act – allowing easy access to bodies for affiliated and favoured medical schools at the cost of the independent schools – is, however, difficult to sustain outside the largest cities.[102] Lay governors were the key force in campaigns for the establishment and financing of voluntary hospitals, largely determining policy, and thus were particularly anxious that hospitals were not seen as granting post-mortems simply to satisfy idle curiosity. It should also be noted that voluntary hospitals in the early nineteenth century were selective in their admissions policy, taking only those cases that were likely to provide recoveries. Children, pregnant women and infectious cases were all excluded, and surgery was very limited in the days before anaesthesia, ensuring that mortality rates were low.

It is tempting to vouch for the paternalistic nature of voluntary hospitals, where the benefactor had a duty to rule but also to provide protection and moral guidance to those in his care. There are obvious regional and metropolitan variations, and much local research is still necessary. In her extensive study of the voluntary hospitals of Wakefield and Huddersfield, Hilary Marland noted the importance of middle-class support for hospitals but a particular lack of clergymen in Yorkshire, and goes on to note the independence of the labouring population as patients.[103] She examined the independence of the workforce in Yorkshire but insists that 'more than many other forms of philanthropy, medical charity gave the donor the chance of personal contract with the recipient, and the opportunity to monitor his or her behaviour and to create a situation of dependency'.[104] In this climate, unauthorized dissection was a risky venture for the voluntary hospital. Even in Edinburgh, a national centre of the new pathological anatomy, a surgeon was sacked in 1759 from the infirmary for conducting an unauthorized post-mortem. He had dissected the head and amputated the legs, claiming that he was practising for an operation to be conducted the following day.[105] In 1718 the apothecary's apprentice at St Thomas's was expelled for keeping bodies from St Saviour's churchyard in his room.[106]

Oxford Hospital Bodies

The records of the Radcliffe Infirmary in Oxford provide an insight into the aspirations and motives of the governors of a provincial hospital and would seem to indicate an institution concerned with its charitable aim towards the sick poor. While the Radcliffe was a growing hospital, the town was, of course, small in comparison with metropolitan centres such as London, Edinburgh and even Manchester. The system of 'turns', which allowed the financial supporters of the hospital to recommend patients, was strong compared to access through casualty areas and doctor-led admission. The new clinical professor was allowed to take his own patients 'as he shall judge expedient for the benefit of the clinical institution' from 1780.[107] By 1816 the rule had been extended to allow honorary physicians and surgeons to recommend six patients each year, with two in-patients at one time.[108] Yet few in-patients were strangers in the town without relatives to bury them.

The hospital, even in the case of unclaimed dead patients from workhouses, appears to have gone to great lengths to bury them: 'Great expense has accrued to the Infirmary by the frequent burials of patients belonging to the several parishes within the city of Oxford'.[109] This becomes particularly apparent after the passage of the Anatomy Act, when the poor law authorities and the infirmary frequently came into conflict over burial responsibility at a time when it was legal to appropriate unclaimed cadavers. The Radcliffe did set aside land for its own cemetery from 1821.[110] A table of interments appears in 1837 and shows a total of forty-five burials for the seven years from 1830 to 1836, but there is no indication of how these bodies were treated.[111]

It is possible that the poor were at first concerned with the possibility of treatment within the Radcliffe. The Radcliffe Infirmary minutes of 1775 report: 'It appears ... the numbers of patients will probably increase every year, as the aversion to the institution ... is entirely worn off'.[112] The anonymity of the metropolis did not exist in Oxford, as a market town dominated by ecclesiastical interests. The influence of the clergy was huge in early nineteenth-century Oxford, with nearly all fellows of the university in holy orders and half the undergraduates aiming to be clergymen (and indeed one-third the sons of clergymen). As influential men in the university, the clergy dominated local charities, including the Radcliffe Infirmary.

The peculiarly ecclesiastical and academic dominance of the Radcliffe Infirmary may have made the institution unusual, and certainly unlike the hospitals of London and other major metropolitan centres. Research certainly suggests that Oxford was generous in terms of numbers of beds to population in the eighteenth century. The Committee of Management and officers of the Radcliffe may have been particularly concerned about the treatment of the poor, certainly in the early days of the infirmary, and could be defined as particularly paternalistic in behaviour.

The clergy in Oxford were often major landowners and magistrates as well as prominent citizens through the university and administrators and educators in all the local charities and institutions. They taught and supervised the poor, and in return they took their duty to protect the poor seriously. The presence of large numbers of clergymen made the city more generous than towns of similar size and structure. This theme is revisited in subsequent chapters. My research on the use of the dead would indicate that the size and peculiar social structure of Oxford ensured that the Radcliffe Infirmary retained its paternalistic ideal over the lives and deaths of the poor. This protection continued even after the Anatomy Act, which gave many institutions an added impetus for the dissection of deceased patients. This ideal may have been common to other market town infirmaries but is less obvious in larger centres. The poor of Oxford, along with the vast majority of the population, abhorred the thought of dissection, and at the Radcliffe Infirmary they were largely protected from this fate. The likelihood of limited post-mortem is, however, impossible to ascertain.

Manchester Hospital Bodies

The evidence for Manchester hospital bodies is less well preserved than that for Oxford, but there are a few interesting cases worth investigating. As noted previously, Thomas Fawdington, house surgeon of the Manchester Infirmary in 1817, was disciplined for opening the body of a girl without parental or hospital permission.[113] Fawdington undertook a post-mortem on a patient at the Eye Institution in 1824, and this examination is well documented because Fawdington published his findings, with illustrations. This operation was not simply a limited post-mortem to ascertain cause of death, but seems to have been a thorough dissection of the eyes, liver, kidneys, lungs, ileum and heart.[114] It is not known whether there was permission for the post-mortem. The catalogues of the Jordan and Fawdington anatomy museums certainly illustrate that body parts were retained for research. There is, however, no means of determining the number of hospital post-mortems before the end of the nineteenth century in most hospitals. The evidence is scarce for Manchester beyond the few examples in the Fawdington and Jordan museum catalogues and the infirmary minutes.

There was some working-class hostility towards the hospitals in Manchester around 1819. The Irish community found the infirmary a particular threat, and antipathy was increased in the aftermath of Peterloo with rumours that the hospital refused treatment to a victim of the riot. In 1828 thirteen-year-old Mary Williamson embroidered a sampler of Manchester Infirmary with the words:

Here too the sick their final doom receive
Here brought amid the scenes of grief to grieve
Where the loud groans from some sad chambers flow
Mix'd with the clamours of the crowd below.[115]

There is, however, no evidence of any lasting antipathy to the voluntary hospitals of Manchester or Oxford and certainly nothing to suggest that post-mortem or dissection was a particular fear among the patients, except at times of particular working-class anxiety. The lack of evidence certainly supports this position. It is important to examine the impact of the additional stress on the relationship between hospital doctors and patients and relatives at the time of the cholera outbreak, covered in the next chapter.

Public Attitudes to Dissection

There has been much work done on the public revulsion towards bodysnatching and dissection, and historians have been able to discern distinct strands of fear. A particular problem for the anatomists in improving supply was the constant link in the public mind between dissection and punishment, as the procedure was reserved in legal terms as the final penalty for murderers, the worst of offenders. Much of the debate conducted in the medical press focused on this issue, with medical commentators concerned that supply would never be improved until this connection was severed. Yet there must have been a more fundamental revulsion towards dissection based on strongly held beliefs about the sanctity of the body, as the gallows crowd, even after the Murder Act, expressed disapproval of the final indignity.

Respect for the body and its treatment after death is not a straightforward issue. Some prisoners were certainly prepared to sell their own bodies for the cost of hanging clothes or other expenses. There is much evidence to suggest, however, that keen attention to the proper forms of burial was believed to be required to ensure the final peaceful rest of the deceased. The dissection of the dead contributed to the final humiliation of the prisoner, and this connection with the gallows added to the abhorrence of dissection within the general population. At an introductory lecture at Surgeons Hall in 1759, the surgeon Mr Tate spoke over the body of Richard Lamb:

> And it being well known, in how great horror dissection was held by almost all mankind, more especially the lower class, as the most harden'd villains, tho' they braved death, still shuddered at the thoughts of being made an Otomy (as they called it).[116]

The removal of murderers as a source of cadavers was a central issue for the medical men calling years later for the passing of the Anatomy Act. The *Lancet* reported on a meeting of the London Medical Society in 1828 where it was observed that 'so long as the present clause remains condemning the murderer to dissection, the public will never consent to the appropriation even of unclaimed bodies to anatomical purposes'.[117] *Jackson's Oxford Journal* reported that the use of criminal bodies for dissection was detrimental to the development of anatomy, 'since it affords only an atom of supply to the demands of teachers, whilst it feeds the prejudice of ignorant persons by implying that dissection is the most suitable punishment for the worst of crimes'.[118] The belief by a large part of the population in the sanctity of the body after death is revealed by the fact that the body's desecration was used as the ultimate punishment within the Murder Act.

Foremost in the public mind, within all ranks of society, was a dread of dissection due to basic Christian doctrine. Although most people understood that the body rotted after death, dismemberment and dispersal destroyed the final hope of the reunification of the soul and body on the Day of Judgement. The standard theological view was that:

> The majority of the faithful would sleep in their graves until on Judgement Day the Spirit of God would breathe life into their bones, and the voice of Christ would order Death to release its grip and the bonds of corruption to fall away.[119]

Under the punishment of dissection, there was no final resting place for the body, as it was mutilated and dispersed into anatomical collections. Doctors, and surgeons in particular, were tainted by their work in dissection and their link with the resurrection men, as the great bulk of the population felt a disgust at bodysnatching based on 'a *shared* conception of respect for the dead and of a shared *sense* of vulnerability to grave-robbery'.[120] John Doherty railed against the trade and demanded

> the complete exposure of every circumstance and person who may be in any way connected with, or aiding in, the horrid and revolting traffic in human flesh, which is now so extensively and daringly carried on in this country, under the specious mask of promoting medical knowledge.[121]

Post-mortem care of the body was therefore extremely important for all social classes at the beginning of the nineteenth century. It was still common for a corpse to be properly laid out and washed and to remain in a coffin at home, closely watched until the funeral, providing solace for those surviving the deceased. Despite the growing secularization of society during the nineteenth century, the sanctity of the grave remained a major tenet of faith, providing for resurrection and reunification with loved ones. The current-day disconnection with the corpse, and our overriding concern for the disposal of the body quickly to avoid sanitary problems, blinds us to the centrality of the body in the death and funeral rituals of the past. Richardson makes a study of funeral invitations in the eighteenth century, in which mourners are asked 'to *accompany the corpse* of the dead person, rather than merely to attend the funeral',[122] thereby providing protection. The surgeon G. A. Walker wrote that 'decently to dispose of the dead, and vigilantly to secure their remains from violation, are among the first duties of society'.[123]

The status of the grave and the provision of a decent funeral preserved the remains for eternity but was also a sign of respectability in a society which recognized that even death had become a commercial business, dividing the successful from those guilty of poverty and failure. While all classes were subject to the threat of bodysnatching, the poor in mass shallow graves and flimsy coffins were most at risk. Wealthy citizens could go to great lengths to protect their bodies from the anatomists, investing in lead coffins and mort-safes as well as various chemical preparations, including:

> A mixture of percussion powder and gunpowder, placed on a wire in the inside of the coffin, to explode on its being opened, has been resorted to. This will retain its explosive power for a month, in which time the corpse will be generally unfit for dissection.[124]

The Reverend J. Scholefield, who practised as an unqualified doctor and was the first minister of the Round Chapel in Every Street, Manchester, advertised safety tombs for purchase.[125] Such extreme measures were unusual, yet they do illustrate concern within the populace.

The rise of the commercial cemetery companies can be viewed in part as a response to concerns over dissection. It was a strong motive in the planning of the General Cemetery of All Souls at Kensal Green, where 'graves should be inviolate, and various gadgets were proposed to ensure the safety of the new cemetery companies' clients' bodies until they had decomposed sufficiently to be useless for dissection'.[126] There were two key factors in the establishment of private cemetery companies: a politically strong nonconformist community who rejected Anglican burial practice; and vitally, a desire to protect the sanctity of the body from body-snatchers. A spoof prospectus for a private cemetery company from 1825 illustrates public opinion of anatomists and the grave. It comes from the 'Life, Death, Burial and Resurrection Company':

> To rob Death of its Terrors, and make it delightful,
> To give up your breath and abolish the frightful
> Old custom of lying defunct in your shroud,
> Surrounded by relatives sobbing aloud ...
> A diversified, soothing, commixture of trees,
> Umbrageous, and fann'd by the perfumed breeze,
> With alcoves, and bowers, and fish-ponds, and shrubs,
> Select, as in life, from intrusion of scrubs.[127]

'Scrubs' was a disparaging term for surgeons. The company was 'supported by Lord Graves and President Coffin, eminent physicians, members of the College of Surgeons'. The very first private cemetery company was started in Manchester in 1820, and the Liverpool necropolis of 1825 promised 'entire security against trespassers of any kind'.[128]

Of course these measures only benefited the wealthier classes, leaving the poor more vulnerable to snatching from cheaper graves. The pauper funeral was to be feared, particularly as standards of post-mortem care largely deteriorated in the nineteenth century, with parishes increasingly anxious to keep costs down. The research on Oxford suggests that there was concern over maintaining a high standard of pauper funeral, but as most of it relates to the period after 1832, it is examined in the following two chapters. The Manchester research certainly suggests that there were mass graves for the poor and that these could be particularly vulnerable. The bodysnatching case reported by the *Manchester Guardian* on 21 February 1824 illustrates this point:

> The place from which they were stolen is a large grave, calculated to contain from twenty to thirty coffins, and was left with a covering of boards only, until the requisite number were deposited. Of course this rendered it easy to remove the bodies, without leaving any traces which would excite suspicion.[129]

While there were obviously gradations of pauper funeral, with a scale of charges and services, there can be no doubt that the Manchester poor were often placed in common graves. Engels wrote in 1845 of a desolate pauper burial ground in Manchester where 'the poor are dumped into the earth like infected cattle'.[130]

In whatever manner the majority of paupers were buried in Manchester, there was certainly public concern over the treatment of the dead body in the grave. Much has been made of the fear of workhouse anatomizing after 1832, but Manchester witnessed public concern over the fate of workhouse paupers as early as 1820:

> A great uproar is occasioned in Manchester by bodies being stolen out of the burying ground adjoining the Manchester workhouse there is often much said also of paupers dying in the workhouse and more so in this town because there is a door communicating from the churchyard to the workhouse gardens and through which paupers are daily carried to be buried.[131]

The author of *The Trial of John Eaton* in Manchester accepted that:

> Anatomical science cannot be cultivated with success, without dissection ... but it may be questioned whether the advantages obtained by the present method of procuring subjects for this purpose, counterbalance the dreadful mental agonies which are inflicted on the living.[132]

His concern was with the grief of the living over the desecration of the grave. The author went on to champion the right of the poor to dispose of what little property they had as they wished, including their relatives:

> The poor man ought not to be defrauded of his property, dismal as it is, nor of his right to the disposal of his own relative, as dear to himself as the body of a prince deposited in a costly mausoleum, erected at the expense of a nation, is to a monarch.[133]

The document advised on the best means for protecting bodies and called for better security of all burial grounds and the crime of resurrection to be made a felony offence applicable to '*all the parties* concerned', thereby demanding punishment for the receiving anatomists.[134]

Popular Attitudes and Responses

Apart from concerns over the unification of the body and soul, there is ample evidence of public disquiet over the treatment of the body at post-mortem by unscrupulous medical men. At a time when the social status of doctors, especially surgeons, was marginal, there was little belief in the professional detachment of the medical man. Thomas Rowlandson's painting *The Persevering Surgeon* depicts a beautiful naked young woman under the knife of a somewhat debauched practitioner with raised knife.[135] Other paintings followed this theme of medical sexual prurience in death, including *The Dissection* of 1780, which pictured anatomists gazing at and stroking the leg of a recently dissected and naked female body. The *Times* reported on the fear of a female relative 'subjected to the gaze of lads learning to use the incision knife'.[136]

The idea of premature anatomizing was used with much success by Edward Ravenscroft in his play *The Anatomist*, first performed in 1696 and in the London repertoire regularly until the 1790s. The farce concerns itself with young lovers, clever servants, mistaken identities and an inept doctor attempting to dissect a living body that gets up and runs away. The doctor's wife says, 'I have heard of such strange things: I warrant the poor man was hang'd wrongfully'.[137] Although a farce, the play touches on contemporary fears over dissection as well as condemning medical men for their poor therapeutic practice and race for status.

The evidence regarding public acceptance of dissection is confused, not helped by the failure of contemporary commentators and writers to discern a distinction between dissection and post-mortem. There is some evidence that there was a limited acceptance of the private post-mortem in Georgian society, with some family requests. However, these appear to be rare and confined to the upper echelons of society. John Hunter conducted post-mortems on the president of the Royal Society and the prime minister, among many others. Some so-called dissections may have been more limited autopsies conducted in order to discover the causes of death, or given the nature of the anatomist concerned, more extensive dissections without the full awareness of any surviving family.[138] Famously, Jeremy Bentham in 1832 and Richard Carlile in 1843 were dissected on their own wishes. However, even the legal requirement for post-mortem examinations conducted through the auspices of coroner's court was a highly sensitive issue. The *Times* reminded its readers that 'the loss of one's relation is distressing enough without (unless occasion should absolutely require it) an additional harrowing of the feelings by the coroner's inquest, and, perhaps, the application of the knife'.[139]

Thomas Wakley, who had been to some extent a sympathizer for the poor over the passing of the Anatomy Act, was the subject of public criticism for ordering greater numbers of post-mortems after he became Middlesex coroner in 1839. Under the headline 'Wholesale Post-Mortem Examinations', the *Morning Herald* reported that Wakley had a '*predilection* for dissecting' and 'mangling *without reasonable motive*'.[140] The increase in post-mortem activity was very gradual through the nineteenth century, and Wakley's efforts to increase rates were largely thwarted. There is very little evidence that the poor regarded dissection, legal or otherwise, with anything other than horror, particularly after the 1751 Murder Act.

Not only were the poor at risk of a pauper funeral leading to a possible dissection, but murder could become the ultimate penalty for poverty. The well-publicized trials of murderers Burke and Hare in Edinburgh and Bishop and Williams in London were a clear illustration to the poor in Manchester and Oxford of their vulnerability and impotence against an increasingly hostile ruling class. Historians have, however, found it difficult to discern any particular concern with bodysnatching and dissection from the poor within a time of particular volatility in the industrial and agricultural regions of England. This social instability is itself the subject of much debate.

There is some evidence that the fear of bodysnatching was part of and became subsumed within a wider social protest that arose out of the increasingly desperate situation of agricultural labourers who perceived an assault by the ruling gentry, and small farmers rejecting the traditional paternalistic role for a relationship based purely on market values. There was a spate of Swing disturbances in Oxfordshire, starting with threatening letters in Henley in November 1830 citing low agricultural wages and a link with enclosure at Otmoor in August of that year. The attempt at enclosure by Thomas Newton at Benson led to a spate of 'Swing-type' machine breaking at Ewelme, Rofford, Burcot and Little Milton, also in November 1830.[141]

Swing riots were motivated by a multiplicity of issues such as 'work, wages, poor relief, the use of machinery and the role of rural elites'.[142] It is likely that the Otmoor disturbances were the result of several grievances. The *Oxford University and City Herald* reported that the extensive moorland of Otmoor, northeast of Oxford, could yield substantial profits for small farmers in terms of summer pasturage; but the 'greatest benefit was reaped by the cottagers, many of whom turned out large numbers of geese, to which the coarse aquatic sward was well suited', and they 'thereby brought up their families in comparative plenty'.[143] There were proposals to enclose the land from 1801, but the measure gained momentum from around 1830 when attitudes to the poor had hardened. The same newspaper wrote: 'God did not create the earth to lye waste for feeding a few geese, but to be cultivated by man in the sweat of his brow'.[144] On 6 September 1830 a crowd gathered on Otmoor and tore down enclosures. Sixty-six people were taken and the Riot Act read, with twenty-five released and forty-one sent for trial at Oxford on the orders of the Reverend Vaughan Thomas. The prisoners were then liberated by an angry crowd. The prosecution papers report that:

> On passing through St Giles's (where an immense number of persons had assembled to enjoy the festivities of a Fair similar to that of St Bartholemew) the military were attacked in every direction; brickbats, stones and bludgeons were hurled at them without mercy.[145]

Enclosure was the key to the outbreaks of violence associated with Otmoor from 1830 until 1835, with a large number of small farmers and respectable citizens rioting. The authorities were particularly outraged by this, as illustrated in the case notes: 'The defendants are not of the lowest orders in life – and have consequently broken the duty they owe to society in setting an example of obedience to the laws to their inferiors'.[146] Other issues were at stake; Philip Green, chimney sweep, rioter and admirer of William Cobbett, addressed the magistrates in 1830 after several of the rioters were re-arrested:

> They had been oppressed long enough and we will bear it no longer, great changes were taking place in other parts of the world and there must be a change here – there was plenty of money in the country if it was equally distributed – the rich have had it their way long enough, and now it is our turn – The machines must come down and every man ought to have two shillings a day.[147]

On September 1831 there was a further attempt to raise a rate to expand enclosure on Otmoor. As a matter of course, the policeman Henry Drake was to affix notices on the relevant village church doors. A crowd of around fifty labourers attempted to prevent this, shouting, 'damn the body-snatchers, if they attempt to pass we'll toss them into the water'.[148] Bodysnatching and dissection was an issue, albeit a minor one in the face of greater assaults upon traditional livelihoods. The disturbance at Otmoor would certainly support Lawrence's contention that 'fears about grave robbing, or about ending up under a student's knife after dying in hospital ... achieved articulation when they encapsulated particularly timely concerns about poverty, powerlessness and the instability of the social order'.[149]

The poor of Oxfordshire were motivated to riot over the issue of enclosure in the early nineteenth century when the perceived bonds of local agricultural society were under threat. Bound up with this focus on enclosure was a multitude of concerns, including the minor anxiety over bodysnatching and anatomy. There would seem to have been little risk of bodysnatching and dissection around Oxford, despite the existence of an early medical (and more specifically) anatomy school, due to the size and ecclesiastical nature of the university-dominated town. The poor of Manchester did not feel moved to protest against anatomy until presented with direct evidence of mutilation during the furore of the cholera outbreak, and this is examined in Chapter 3.

Conclusion

There is overwhelming evidence to support the contention that legal bodies were an inadequate source of material for the growing number of anatomists around the country. There seems to have been something of a mania for dissecting among students in the eighteenth and nineteenth centuries and no effective way of preserving cadavers, yet few bodies were available to any anatomists even after the 1752 Murder Act. There is, however, a need for further regional studies to adjust the existing scholarship. Surgeons and physicians in Manchester and Oxford certainly appear to have received few legal bodies, particularly in Manchester, where anatomy teaching was based in private schools that gave them little authority at the gallows. Oxford University was entitled to receive bodies from the hangman, but there were very few murderers in the vicinity resulting in a small number of cadavers for teaching purposes.

There is some evidence that doctors in both cities attempted to use illicit means to gain a supply, with far greater success achieved in Manchester. Bodysnatching was not a viable option for Oxford, with its very small population and the political and social dominance of the clerically trained university elite. Indeed, the evidence suggests that bodysnatching was not a major source of bodies outside major centres such as London and possibly, to some extent, Manchester. There is of course evidence presented here that large towns such as London and Manchester may have assisted other locations through a trade in corpses, and this is a fruitful area for further research.

Prior to 1832 dissection was feared, and it was common knowledge that the poorer grave was at greater risk of bodysnatching and dissection. That fear was based on complex personal feelings about the body as well as concern over the resurrection of the body and soul, which was considered to be unlikely if body parts were dispersed into anatomical collections. Antipathy to dissection was also caused by the link in the public imagination with punishment at the gallows, under the 1752 Murder Act. There is some evidence to suggest that attitudes to the more limited post-mortem hardened at the same time, and the procedure was, at best, treated with suspicion.

The dearth of subjects to a newly confident and expanding professional group of anatomists was one reason for the institution of the 1828 Select Committee on Anatomy. The profession needed to distance itself from the activities of the resurrection men, which resulted in public condemnation and ridicule, but the major catalyst was the indictment of medical men in a case of bodysnatching and the risk of actual imprisonment. The Bill was finally passed in 1832 after the discovery of a second set of 'burkers'. The passage of the legislation and its effect upon the poor of Oxford and Manchester is the subject of the following chapter.

3 THE ANATOMY ACT AND THE POOR

This book has so far examined the level of public concern over anatomy and dissection before the passing of the Anatomy Act and the extent of bodysnatching activity in Oxford and Manchester. While the poor were most at risk from the bodysnatcher, all classes of society were affected by the risk of anatomization. The 1832 Anatomy Act went a step further, specifically targeting the poor alone for dissection by allowing the so-called unclaimed bodies of those dying in workhouses and other public institutions to be used by licensed anatomists. The present chapter examines, firstly, the passing of the Anatomy Act, including the circumstances that finally galvanized Parliament into action. Richardson has examined the Select Committee on Anatomy in her groundbreaking work, and so this chapter focuses on aspects of this institution not detailed by Richardson, and particularly when its proceedings cast light upon anatomy in Manchester and Oxford. The research examines opinions and actions in Parliament, through Hansard, around the passing of the Act, an area that has been somewhat neglected by historians of the Anatomy Act.

It is also necessary to investigate the further demonstrations of public disquiet that took place during and immediately after the passing of the Anatomy Act. The previous chapter commenced the discussion of a problem in discerning any particular public concern over the passing of the Act, but there is in fact much evidence in contemporary local newspapers of public fears over 'burking', or murder for the purpose of dissection, particularly in Manchester. Chapter 2 argued that bodysnatching fears could be bound up with public disorder, including enclosure riots, and much of the public concern was masked by the tumult over the passing of the Reform Act and the cholera outbreak of 1831–2. Manchester and other regional centres certainly experienced riots that focused directly on the anatomy school and unauthorized dissection. The fear of dissection during the cholera outbreak, despite the protestations of medical men, was real and justified.

The passing of the Anatomy Act was not covered in detail by contemporary newspapers, and regrettably much of the parliamentary record does not survive. As with the Otmoor disturbance discussed in the previous chapter, the public disquiet over anatomy and dissection in 1832 can often only be discerned in contemporaneous public fears, notably over cholera and the Reform Act. The furore arising around the arrival of cholera initially masks fear over anatomization in the population, but these can ultimately be discerned within cholera riots.

Catalysts for Legislation – Conviction of Doctors and the Select Committee on Anatomy

The growing number of medical students, largely at the private anatomy schools, and the accompanying difficulty of procuring sufficient bodies led to increasingly strident calls for legislative regulation. Doctors had long been aware that their connection with bodysnatchers was damaging to their claims of respectability, and the legal use of prisoners' bodies ensured that the notion of dissection was a punishment in the public perception.

The campaign for legislative change led by medical men took on a sense of urgency when the respectability of the profession was under greater threat, and the government then acted to protect medical interests.[1] There were two elements to this: firstly, the growing likelihood of a doctor being imprisoned for bodysnatching; and secondly, the linking of medical men with murder after the discovery of a gang of murderers or 'burkers' in London, confirming fears that the rewards of bodysnatching would ultimately lead to the crime of murder. In 1823 five medical students from Bristol were charged with assault while exhuming bodies, although the case against them was later dropped. In March 1827 John Davis, a medical student, and William Blundell, dispensary attendant and surgeon-apothecary, were convicted of receiving the body of Jane Fairclough from bodysnatchers in Warrington and were duly fined. The judge in the case at Lancaster Assizes pronounced words of concern to every anatomist in the country:

> The only bodies legally liable to dissection in this country were those of persons executed for murder. However necessary it might be, for the purposes of humanity and science that these things should be done, yet as long as the law remained as it was at present, the disinterment of bodies for dissection was an offence liable to punishment.[2]

Manchester's leading anatomist, Joseph Jordan, noted the problem for the dissector:

> You were required to understand your profession, but you were utterly forbidden to dissect, you had no means of obtaining subjects, you were prosecuted if you robbed church-yards. Here you were: the public and the Legislative demanding from you a knowledge of your profession, and yet the law utterly prevented you obtaining that knowledge.[3]

The Select Committee to Inquire into the Manner of Obtaining Subjects for Dissection in the Schools of Anatomy, and into the State of the Law Affecting the Persons Employed in Obtaining or Dissecting Bodies was set up and chaired by Henry Warburton MP in the spring of 1828. The institution of the Select Committee was not a result of the murdering activities of Burke and Hare, but was rather due to the attempted prosecution of medical men, and the final Report from the Select Committee contains a long extract from the Warrington bodysnatchers case heard at the 1828 spring assizes in Lancaster, demonstrating the level of concern from legislators and elite medical men.[4] Despite the fact that the instances of possible prosecution of doctors took place solely in the provinces, the Select Committee drew every single witness from the London, Edinburgh and Dublin medical establishment. Thomas Wakley was the only witness to champion the teaching of anatomy in the provinces, specifically Manchester.[5] Edmund Balfour, secretary to the Royal College of Surgeons, criticized the teaching available in the regions and noted the damage done in the Warrington case: 'It has been found impossible to teach anatomy in the country; and I need not remind this committee of the uproar in which individuals have involved themselves in attempting to teach anatomy in the country'.[6]

Much of the evidence presented to the Committee focused on the centrality of anatomy to the education of doctors and the shortage of cadavers. Benjamin Brodie (senior surgeon at St George's and personal surgeon to the king) felt that each student should have to dissect five bodies over the course of his training;[7] and during his extensive evidence, Sir Astley Cooper stated that 'without dissection there can be no anatomy, and that anatomy is our polar star, for, without anatomy a surgeon can do nothing, certainly nothing well'.[8] Dr Southwood Smith, lecturer in physiology at the Webb Street School and author of *The Use of the Dead to the Living*, gave evidence insisting that anyone going on to practise as a surgeon should dissect at least nine or ten bodies.[9] William Lawrence, surgeon at St Bartholemew's Hospital, felt that each student should have access to three or four bodies during each year of training.[10] John Abernethy (1764–1831), surgeon to St Bartholemew's and lecturer in anatomy and surgery, declared:

> It is of the highest importance to the public; nothing in life, I believe, that can be considered as more important; it is the foundation of all medical knowledge is not merely requisite in order that we may perform operations successfully, but it is the foundation of physiology; and the knowledge of the structure and functions of the organs and parts of the body is the sole source of our knowledge of disease.[11]

After pages of such evidence, the final report accepted the argument over anatomy and queried the Society of Apothecaries' lack of insistence upon dissection for the licence to practise as a general practitioner when this branch of the profession supposedly had to act as surgeons in the provinces.[12] Little consideration was given to the reality that the provincial general practitioner had little need for knowledge of detailed anatomy. By this time, anatomy was accepted as the pre-eminent medical discipline.

The Committee was extremely concerned over the sentencing of doctors in cases of bodysnatching, and it asked witnesses, including Sir Astley Cooper, about their awareness of the law. Sir Astley apparently believed that the hated bodysnatchers would shoulder all the guilt over exhumation:

> Question: Have the gentlemen of the profession been aware that the only bodies legally liable to dissection in this country were the bodies of those persons who have been executed for murder? Answer: We did not consider, until of late, that it was a misdemeanour to have a body in our possession.[13]

John Watson, secretary to the Court of Examiners at the Society of Apothecaries, was asked whether the Society was aware that bodysnatching was a misdemeanour. Unlike Sir Astley Cooper, Watson admitted that the Society was quite aware of this and had therefore never demanded dissection as an examined skill for the licence to practise.[14]

All the medical witnesses stressed the undesirability of dealing with bodysnatchers in an effort to promote their own respectability and distance themselves from the shame of the trade. Sir Astley Cooper told the Select Committee that the resurrectionists were:

> The lowest dregs of degradation ... there is no crime they would not commit, and, as to myself, if they should imagine that I would make a good subject, they really would not have the smallest scruple, if they could do the thing undiscovered, to make a subject of me.[15]

In fact, Cooper also implicated the respectable medical man with the trade in the same evidence, by boasting that he could obtain any body he chose: 'for there is no person, let his situation in life be what it may, whom, if I were disposed to dissect, I could not obtain'.[16]

The Select Committee examined the opinions of twenty-nine witnesses on the use of prisoners' bodies. Twenty-three of them said that the use of murderers' bodies was damaging in the public mind. Sir Astley Cooper stated, 'the law enforcing the dissection of murderers is the greatest stigma on anatomy which it receives, and is extremely injurious to science'.[17] Sir Benjamin Brodie was asked, 'you are of the opinion, therefore, that tolerating exhumation, you are in fact tolerating the existence of a set of the most depraved men in society?' He answered, 'certainly, theirs must be a great school of vice'.[18] He proclaimed that bodysnatchers were 'as bad as any in society'.[19] John Abernethy said 'they are a very bad set of men'.[20] J. H. Green (1791–1863), surgeon at St Thomas's and teacher of anatomy, was asked:

Is it not a distressing thing to a gentleman of character and education to be obliged to have recourse to persons of this description for obtaining the necessary means of giving instruction to their pupils? Certainly, it really made me for some years, when I had the immediate conducting of the business, I may say quite unhappy.[21]

Richard Grainger (1801–65)[22] agreed that 'they are certainly the worst part of society'.[23] None of the medical men acknowledged the valuable role professional bodysnatchers had played in the success of their anatomical work or ever admitted the roles doctors and medical students may have played in exhumation. Certainly in the provinces, medical men, with their own claims to professional respectability, were not above resurrection activities, as illustrated in the Warrington court case.

The Manchester surgeon and teacher Thomas Turner suggested three 'unobjectionable' solutions to the shortage of bodies in his letter to Henry Warburton, which was appended to the final Select Committee report. In common with most witnesses, Turner favoured the use of the 'unclaimed' as well as imports from Ireland and the continent. Unlike most of those examined, Turner wished to retain the executed from Lancaster, but these could only be 'an auxiliary source'.[24] The key point of Turner's solution was supported by most witnesses to the Committee, as the final report illustrated:

It is the opinion of almost all the witnesses ... that the bodies of those who during life have been maintained at the public charge, and who die in workhouses, hospitals, and other charitable institutions, should if not claimed by next of kin within a certain time after death, be given up, under proper regulations, to the anatomist; and some of the witnesses would extend the same rule to the unclaimed bodies of those who die in prison, penitentiaries, and other places of confinement.[25]

Witnesses were at pains to assure the Committee members that remains were treated with respect: 'Is it the practice to bury the remains? Yes, the remains are buried'.[26] Only George Guthrie, in his letter, was clear that this could not possibly mean whole-body burial, as parts would be kept for anatomical preparations.[27]

The Committee made no effort to discern the attitude of poor people at risk of dying in institutions beyond questioning medical men about hospital admission. Brodie was questioned at length on this matter, and he stated that he was not aware of any 'disinclination on the part of the poor to gain admission to those hospitals which have dissecting establishments attached to them'.[28] He went on to say that he did not see much difference between dissection and postmortem and claimed that the dislike of both was on the decrease:

The more people's minds are familiarized to dissection, the less they think of it. Those who live in the neighbourhood of an anatomical school think nothing about it; I remember some years ago, it so happened that several bodies, I believe as many as ten, were brought in to the dissecting room in Windmill-Street in the middle of the day;

and many persons in the street must have known it, and it did not excite the smallest attention among them, they were accustomed to it.[29]

Abernethy agreed that the possibility of dissection did not affect hospital admissions: 'there is a hospital in this town where the poor know that most of the bodies are dissected, and yet applications for admission there are as numerous as in other hospitals'.[30] Guthrie supported this position in a letter to the Secretary of State regarding the Select Committee:

> It has been proved that where dissecting establishments have been attached to hospitals, they have not had the slightest influence in diminishing the number of applications for admission; although it is the common opinion of the poor, that all who die without friends are regularly dissected in them.[31]

Unless social mores were directly offended by blatant disregard for appearances, the anatomy teachers in London were acknowledged and then largely ignored. Guthrie stated that there was no concern over dissecting establishments unless 'the place becomes offensive'. John Hunter undertook post-mortems on the great and the good, but alongside these he also performed post-mortems requested by grieving families, including examinations upon infants. There is supporting material for this from Manchester and Oxford considered later in this chapter and in Chapter 2; yet coronial post-mortems were often the subject of much concern, and this is examined in Chapter 5.

There was no evidence given to the Committee from the English universities, but several provincial medical men wrote letters to the Committee, and these were included in the report. Thomas Turner's letter from Manchester, written on 30 April 1828 and complaining of the recent cadaver shortage, appears in the appendices:

> I have delivered lectures on anatomy and physiology for the last six years, and during the first three or four seasons I was tolerably well supplied ... but of late we have had extreme difficulty in obtaining subjects.[32]

Turner protested over high prices resulting in only forty or fifty bodies available to the seventy or eighty medical students at the two main anatomy schools in Manchester. The final report upheld the opinion of the bulk of the witnesses, the anatomy teachers, yet insisted that the use of unclaimed bodies was of particular interest to the poor and middle classes as these sections of the population tended to consult the more poorly educated general practitioners:

> To neglect the practice of dissection, would lead to the greatest aggravation of human misery; since anatomy, if not learned by that practice, must be learned by mangling the living. Though all classes are deeply interested in affording protection to the study

of anatomy, yet the poor and middle classes are the most so; they will be the most benefited by promoting it, and the principal sufferers by discouraging it.[33]

The Committee's report was submitted to the House of Commons on 22 July 1828, well before the discovery that the natural development of the trade in bodies was murder. The first attempt to pass an Anatomy Act was introduced in March 1829, six weeks after the execution of William Burke.[34] There was little organized opposition to the Bill in the Commons, although several voices of dissent declaimed loudly and the *London Medical Gazette* objected to the 'ravings of Hunt and Cobbett'. The *Gazette*, in common with much of the medical press, could see no argument over the use of 'unclaimed' bodies.

> How astonishing it is that men should be found blind, infatuated and bigoted enough, not to suffer that the bodies of those who have no friends whose feelings can be outraged, should be dissected, rather than that the whole community be under the dread of exhumation, and the graves of all exposed to the visit of the ruffian exhumator.[35]

As demonstrated in the previous chapter, Thomas Wakley, surgeon and editor of the *Lancet*, promoted the elevation of anatomy and dissection in medical teaching, but he was one medical voice largely opposed to the first Anatomy Bill. He termed it 'the Midnight Bill, or the Murderers' Bill, or the Fools' Bill; for a blacker measure, never received the sanction of the "Collective Wisdom".[36] Wakley was in this instance protesting over the likelihood of an Act increasing the power of the Royal College of Surgeons in anatomical teaching. However, Wakley also objected to the focus on pauper bodies, which was 'founded on the cruelty of making an arbitrary disposition of the bodies of the poor, after their lives shall have been worn out in the service of their task masters'. He demanded that '*all* unclaimed bodies should be appropriated, without reference to the rank or wealth of the deceased'.[37]

For those who objected to the use of pauper bodies, alternative sources were difficult to find. Wakley favoured the use of all unclaimed bodies but recognized that this would still fall disproportionately on the poor. He also made attempts to improve the climate for bequests, which would be difficult for some time to come due to the link between dissection and punishment in the public mind. Others sought to avoid the use of workhouse poor by increasing the connection with convicts. One writer to the *Lancet* noted that the great mortality of the floating prison hulks could provide many bodies, as so few were claimed by relatives.[38]

The Anatomy Bill failed in the Lords in June 1829, when aristocrats and clergymen in the House of Lords defended the rights of the poor to a safe burial. Elements of the medical profession had also objected to the Bill, not in its prime intentions but in the detail of the Act's potential administration. Edinburgh University was concerned that there were very few unclaimed bodies in the city.[39] The *London Medical Gazette* articulated a major concern that anatomists risked a fifty-pound fine if bodies were not ultimately buried whole. The *Gazette* complained that this was 'absurd and injurious ... the utmost care could not prevent parts of different bodies being buried as one person'.[40] Despite assurances to the Select Committee, anatomists certainly kept different parts of bodies regularly for museums and teaching purposes, as has already been evidenced in the previous chapter.

'Burking'

On 7 February 1829 the *Oxford University and City Herald* reported on the activities of Burke and Hare. The newspaper called for all medical men to turn their attention to the legislation relating to dissection that was before the Commons: the legislation supported a doctors' petition to Parliament from Norwich and demanded the end of the practice of using prisoners' bodies 'since it affords only an atom of supply to the demands of teachers, whilst it feeds the prejudice of ignorant persons by implying that dissection is the most suitable punishment for the worst of crimes'. The article supported the investigation of imports, encouraging bequests and using 'unknown and unclaimed parties' in order to remove existing temptation to murder.

Burking was discovered in London in November 1831, perpetrated by three men, one a long-standing bodysnatcher.[41] There does not appear to have been any particular reaction to the discovery of 'burking' in Edinburgh and London within the Oxford population, but Manchester newspapers reported on the growing hysteria in their own city. *The Voice of the People* produced an article under the headline 'Mince Pies – Burking Extraordinary':

> The whole of Little Ireland, Oxford Road, was on Wednesday last thrown into a complete uproar by a report getting abroad that another burking establishment, carrying on business to a great extent, had been discovered in the neighbourhood of Little Ireland, from which many a *savoury pie piping hot* had been served to the hungry public.

A dead greyhound, a dead cat and the skeleton of a child had been found at a pie shop run by an old woman, Amelia Anderton, whose son-in-law apparently prepared skeletons for surgeons. After the discovery of murder, all resurrection men and those connected with them could be seen as murderers of the poor. The Manchester pair were taken into custody for their own protection from their neighbours.[42] In February 1831 the same newspaper reported on two constables who stopped a man carrying a heavy parcel in Salford: 'On opening the bundle they found its contents to be a dead pig ... on further enquiry it was found to have been burked'.[43]

The Anatomy Act

The public furore over the discovery of burkers in London and the hardening of attitudes towards the poor in the three years since Warburton's first Anatomy Bill allowed the reintroduction of the Anatomy Act just twelve days after the executions of the London burkers, Bishop and Williams, in December 1831. The legislation was rushed along: by January 1832 the Bill was at the second reading stage, and debate introducing the second reading took place the day after a long session on the Reform Bill.[44] A detailed examination of Hansard illustrates that discussion of the Anatomy Act was often curtailed or even lost within the morass of the debate over the Reform Bill. Mr Robinson of Worcester said that 'he was sure the Bill could not properly be discussed as long as the Reform Bill was before the House and he was determined it should not be passed *pro forma*'.[45] Colonel Sibthorp of Lincoln supported this complaint:

> He protested against proceeding any further with the Bill until it had been carefully discussed, and more information should have been obtained. Here a Bill had been read a first and a second time, and on both occasions, at a late hour, in the night, without any discussion.[46]

Lord William Lennox was hostile to the Anatomy Bill as it was passed. He stated that 'it had been carried through the House in a most disgraceful manner, there rarely being more than forty members present during the discussions concerning it'.[47]

In January 1832 Mr Cresset Pelham of Lincolnshire observed that the Bill was unfairly injurious to the poor, and he stated that he

> was not so impressed with the indispensable necessity of procuring subjects as some other honorary gentlemen appeared to be ... by confining the operation of the Bill, in a great degree, to the poorer classes, it must tend to perpetuate existing prejudices against a practice, which the usage of devoting the bodies of murderers only for the purpose of dissection had invested with the most ignominious associations.[48]

The link between anatomy and punishment was a particular area of concern even for those who wished to utilize unclaimed bodies. Sir Robert Inglis, MP for the University of Oxford, was pleased to note at second reading stage that the use of criminal bodies had been removed from the Bill. There was still, however, 'no provision ... for the decent interment of the remains of those persons who had been the subject of anatomical investigation'. Inglis demonstrated a concern for the bodies of the poor but noted that few bodies were legally available to medical students in the previous year:

> He believed that the science of anatomy could not at present be legally followed. He was satisfied that the study of that science was necessary for the successful practice of medicine, and that, therefore, some means must be taken to remedy the present state of the law.[49]

Inglis supported the use of unclaimed bodies but continued to oppose the use of criminals and even those dying in hospital, as 'it was essential that those whose duty it was to cure should have no interest to kill'. He continued to insist upon the provision of Christian burial and that those expressing antipathy should be spared from dissection.[50]

There were few committed voices of dissent, one of the most vociferous being the radical MP for Preston, Henry Hunt (1773–1835), who had opposed the use of bodies of the poor since 1828 and continued to speak against the re-introduction of the legislation; he promised that he would propose

> An amendment which would oblige every young surgeon, before he handled the knife, to sign an instrument giving up his own body after death for dissection. To any clause which gave up the bodies of the poor and unprotected for dissection he should move an amendment that the bodies of those rich paupers on the Pension List should be given up for the same purpose.[51]

Hunt presented a petition from Lancashire on the 'dead body bill', complaining of the power given to governors in workhouses 'to sell the bodies of the persons who died in those houses; thus making a distinction between the rich and the poor'. Supporters of the Bill objected at the outset to the term 'dead body bill' and reiterated that the purpose of the Bill was to regulate anatomy. Mr O'Connell insisted that the Anatomy Act would be to the advantage of the poor:

> They were more interested than any other class of persons that surgeons in general should have the power of obtaining a scientific education cheaply, and they could not obtain the necessary knowledge without every facility being afforded them of examining the structure of the human body.[52]

The Anatomy Act received royal assent on 1 August 1832, setting up a national inspectorate of anatomy that would authorize the granting of licences to practise anatomy. The provisions of the Act were vague in the extreme, and its discretionary nature allowed for much confusion over the working of the legislation. Eligible bodies were those supposedly unclaimed in public institutions. To avoid anatomization, individuals should have expressed their antipathy to dissection either verbally or in writing, and in the presence of two witnesses. The pronouncement had to take place 'during the illness whereof he died',[53] which obviously made no allowance for sudden death, and there was no compulsion to inform workhouse inmates of this clause. The body had to remain in the institution for at least forty-eight hours after death to allow claimants to come forward, but again with no compulsion to inform relatives or friends of the death within the terms of the Act. There was no definition of who was allowed to claim a body and whether they then became liable for the costs of burial. A certificate of interment from the licensed anatomist had to be received by the Inspector of

Anatomy within six weeks of death. The Act allowing murderers to be dissected was repealed – in future murderers were to be hung in chains or buried within the prison walls.[54] The later working of the Anatomy Act in Oxford and Manchester will be examined in a subsequent chapter. It is now useful to investigate the initial reaction to the legislation and its immediate impact upon the poor, which takes place almost wholly within the tumult surrounding the outbreak of cholera in England in 1832.

Cholera

It is extremely difficult to ascertain workhouse inmates' reactions to the Act and its passage through Parliament, although Richardson has noted several pertinent examples of workhouse disturbances over dissection.[55] Many workhouse records were destroyed on the arrival of the 1948 welfare legislation, and unfortunately this is the case for Manchester and Oxford. As a result, it has been difficult to discern any particular concern over the Anatomy Act in the local populations in Oxford and Manchester, beyond the newspaper coverage of 'burking' fears. The anatomy legislation was inevitably overshadowed by the third Reform Bill, which was introduced to Parliament just three days before the Anatomy Bill.

For much of the public, the Anatomy Act must have evinced feelings of relief as it promised the guarantee of safe burial. Those under threat after 1832 were only those at risk of dying in the workhouse or other public institutions. The framers of the legislation and many doctors believed that only the very poor, 'with no friends' and therefore 'no wish on the subject', would be affected.[56] This section of the population had few opportunities to express their opinions, and newspapers in the two cities usually upheld the attitudes of the medical fraternity. The radical Manchester paper *Poor Man's Advocate* was a notable exception, proclaiming that the Act illustrated that 'not content with the people's toil while living, the rich insist upon having their bodies cut up and mangled when dead'.[57] For these reasons, it is helpful to examine the impact of the 1832 outbreak of cholera in Manchester and Oxford. The disease affected all classes, but the poor were most at risk of the sanitary measures taken by doctors on the new boards of health set up to deal with the public health aspects of the outbreak. This brought the medical men into direct conflict with the local poor while the anatomy legislation was fresh, illustrating deep-seated fears of doctors and anatomy.

The first case of Asiatic cholera was confirmed in Sunderland in October 1831. The government had already responded to the threat of the disease by setting up the Central Board of Health, with a network of local boards instituting highly unpopular public health measures. Dissection was at the heart of fears about cholera, particularly cholera hospitals. During the outbreak, the Gateshead Board of Health reported:

> The common people firmly believe the doctors stupefy their patients with laudanum
> and then hurry them off to the grave while yet alive and that they have dissected living
> bodies; many well-informed people too, think some have been interred alive.[58]

Dissection of cholera bodies certainly took place from the very start of the outbreak. In Sunderland a physician's wife became one of the first victims: 'she had
unwisely been present at the dissection of the nurse who had died in the infirmary'.[59]

The Oxford Board of Health first met in November 1831 and consisted of
the university vice-chancellor, the town mayor and equal representatives from
the city and the university, along with a selection of medical men. Their mor-
alizing attitude to the poor of the city was unlikely to endear the new health
measures to the population of deprived areas and did little to promote the
activities of medical men advocating inspection and removal to new cholera
hospitals: 'The Oxford Board of Health for the third time entreats you to for-
bear and to abstain from all acts of intemperance and imprudence. Beware long
sittings, dancing, revellings, surfeiting, and such like'. The Board advised against
attendance at the popular St Giles's Fair, urging 'caution and remonstrance to all
drunkards and revellers and to the thoughtless and imprudent of both sexes'.[60]
Cholera was a convenient means to preach retribution throughout the country.
The publication *Why are You Afraid of the Cholera?* stated, 'the greater part of
those who have died have been bad, dirty, drunken and idle people'.[61]

John Kidd, professor of medicine at Oxford University during the cholera
outbreak of 1831–2, clearly believed that the local doctors were helping the
poor: 'let there be for the present a community of practice and let the distinc-
tions of medical rank be lost in the common desire to help our fellow creatures
in the common danger'.[62] Nevertheless the disease was a swift killer, and the perceived need to act to prevent the spread of cholera demonstrated to the poor the
insensitivity of the medical men. Doctors could enter any house suspected of
infection with cholera and order cleansing and burning of belongings. Orders
from the Central Board of Health were given for the burial of victims within
twelve hours of death, depriving the families of traditional funerary customs and
causing fear of premature burial and possibly dissection. There is evidence in the
Oxford Board of Health papers of concern over public objection. When Robert Stone died one night, 'Mr Allen thought it would be best to inter his body
and that of Sarah Cheeseman at the same time'. Both bodies were taken by punt
down the canal to the back of the church, 'thereby avoiding any crowd of persons
that might be congregated together in the parish of St Thomas'.[63]

There are no direct references to dissection or post-mortem in the Oxford
Board of Health papers, but on 3 October 1832 Mr Symonds presented to the
Board 'memoirs on the history, nosology, symptoms, prognostics, diagnosis,
post-mortem appearances, pathology, treatment and final causes of cholera'.[64] The

Oxford doctors were particularly unsuccessful in persuading victims of the disease to enter the new cholera hospitals (out of 174 cases, only twenty-four went to the hospital[65]), and the Board resorted to scaremongering: 'Look to Godfrey's Row – look to Bull Street – and learn from their afflictions a lesson profitable to yourselves. Like you, they tarried too long in the midst of disease, and sooner than quit their habitations, many sickened and died.'[66] Oxford surgeons visited Sunderland at the outbreak, and in August 1832 they 'informed the Board that there was the same reluctance to going into the cholera hospital which we experienced – the same unworthy imputations upon the faculty from the ignorant.'[67]

Cholera certainly heightened the unease and mistrust felt about the medical profession and the Anatomy Act in 1832, and this was particularly apparent in Manchester, with direct protests over the suspicion of unauthorized dissection. The papers of the Manchester Board of Health illustrate that the relationship between the poor and the medical men was particularly bad, and that the poor did not trust the actions of doctors within the cholera hospitals. The Manchester Board of Health asked the clergy to give sermons and Sunday schools 'best calculated to remove the present prejudices against the cholera hospitals from the minds of the poorer classes of the community'.[68] A further communication noted that an advertisement was needed to assure the population that the clergy of the collegiate church were still conducting burial services on cholera victims and not simply leaving them to the medical men.[69] Dr Gaulter, Manchester physician, reported on Martha Chorlton of Ancoats: 'upon inspecting her body after death, we then found an encysted tumour in the right lobe of the liver'.[70] He also opened the cobbler Richard Bullock and his two daughters, Martha, eight months, and Jane, three years: 'On inspection, after death' Gaulter found lesions in 'the viscera of the children'. The use of the term 'inspection' is vague and does not give any idea as to the extent of the post-mortem examination. Gaulter believed that the deaths of these three victims were particularly harmful to the reputation of the Knott Mill cholera hospital. The mother of the children had been forced into the cholera hospital by the doctors, and 'the mob which collected at the gates of the hospital loudly accused the doctors of poison, and even of darker crimes'.[71] Gaulter believed that 'the poor of this town never overcame their horror of the cholera hospitals'.[72]

A major riot in Manchester occurred during the epidemic, centred on the cholera hospital and a case of unauthorized dissection. On 8 September 1832 the *Manchester Guardian* reported 'outrage at the Cholera Hospital':

> It is our painful duty this week to record one of those ebullitions of prejudiced feeling on the part of the lower classes against the medical officers of a cholera hospital, from which we had hoped that this town would have continued free.

The head of a child had been removed and replaced with a brick. The crime was only discovered when the grandfather removed the lid of the coffin on collection, as the name inscribed was incorrect. A crowd formed around the grandfather and the headless body was paraded around town, provoking rumours of murder at the hospital in addition to dissection. The Swan Street Hospital was stormed by around 2,000 people, many of whom rescued friends and relations. The cholera van was destroyed, but the hospital was allowed to stand out of respect for the remaining patients. An apothecary, Robert Oldham, was blamed (and indeed, the child's head was found at his lodgings), and he fled. Order was finally restored and the child properly interred, but the *Manchester Guardian* article illustrates the fears of the Board of Health and the suspicion under which doctors operated:

> We understand that an impression prevails in some quarters that the Board of Health first permitted Robert Oldham to affect his escape, and then took out a warrant against him, without any serious intention of causing him to be apprehended. In contradiction of this erroneous notion, we are authorised to state, that no member of the board ever saw Oldham after his guilt was ascertained, or knew where to find him, that the warrant was applied for as soon as possible, and that active measures are taking for his apprehension.[73]

The *Manchester Guardian* was highly critical of the 'ignorant' behaviour of the Manchester crowd despite the reality of the fears of the poor. The Oxford newspaper reported the incident in more measured tones, recognizing the problem for doctors:

> The cries of execration against the doctors were very general ... It is regretted that any of the surgeons should have used any part of the body of a person dying of cholera for surgical purposes, as the antipathy of the lower orders to the cholera hospital has been so great.[74]

The *Poor Man's Advocate* saw the situation from the point of view of the poor. The editor John Doherty, in an article critical of the *Manchester Guardian*, wrote that 'cholera riot [was] no proof of the people's ignorance' and asserted that the poor of Manchester had actually been correct to mistrust doctors in the cholera hospitals.[75] The *Poor Man's Advocate* reported long before the riot that the hospitals were 'a means of removing the poor sick from the sight of their friends so that they may more conveniently be butchered and anatomized by the doctors'.[76] The Central Board of Health was aware of this fear and urged doctors to proceed cautiously 'to avoid discontent'. All dissections were to have relatives' permission.[77] The dissection of the child that was at the heart of the Manchester cholera riot was not, however, an isolated occurrence. Robert Oldham was presented by the Board of Health and the press as a rogue dissector, but the resident surgeon at the Swan Street hospital stated that he regularly examined the 'bodies of those who died in collapse'.[78]

An examination of the cholera riot in the neighbouring city of Liverpool would support the contention that the disease was a convenient vehicle for expressions of anger against bodysnatching, medical men and dissection.[79] *The Liverpool Mercury* reported that 'amongst great numbers of the lower classes in this town the idea is prevalent that the cholera is a mere invention of the medical men to fill their pockets', and that the sufferers were 'victims of experiments while living and subjects for the dissecting knife when dead'.[80] The city was hit very hard by the disease, with 4,977 cases and 1,523 deaths, and the fear of the poor resulted in eight separate riots over ten days in the late spring of 1832. The first riot took place outside the Toxteth Park Cholera Hospital, with shouts of 'bring out the burkers'.[81] Once again the local press criticized the rioters, reporting on 'a most disgraceful instance of combined ignorance, prejudice and folly'.[82] The violence was only quelled by public statements from doctors denying the use of dead bodies and an appeal by the Catholic Church that patients could be visited daily in the cholera hospitals and bodies inspected before burial.[83]

Anatomy Riots

Michael Durey has made a survey of thirty separate riots that took place during the cholera epidemic, illustrating the level of suspicion of doctors and concern over nefarious burial practices. Of these, eight focused the attack on doctors, eight on hospitals and six on churchyards. Burking was mentioned in five, poisoning in eight, dissection in five and burial rights in six.[84] Two further riots in Cambridge and Sheffield are worth considering as they were not sparked by cholera but were a direct attack upon the provisions of the Anatomy Act. Both towns have much in common with Oxford and Manchester. Shortly after the passing of the Act, the need for discretion and secrecy stressed by the Anatomy Inspector was made obvious.[85] In December 1833 the body of a pauper was removed to the Anatomy School at Cambridge University. He had not died in the workhouse but did require a parish coffin and burial. *Jackson's Oxford Journal* reported on the incident, which was the subject of a public meeting: 'On Monday night the mob assembled, forced the Anatomy School, broke the windows, and destroyed some of the skeletons, models and preparations'.[86]

The Inspector of Anatomy, James Somerville, was under the impression that the victim was a baby, and wrote with concern to Professor Clark:

> It is with great concern that I see in the Times of this morning, an allusion to some riotous proceedings at Cambridge, in reference to the removal of a baby to the school of anatomy. You will readily believe that the greatest anxiety prevails at the Home Office to know the particulars and I shall feel greatly obliged by any statement which you may think it advisable to make for the information of Lord Melbourne.[87]

The Home Office responded with equal concern and annoyance: 'the parish authorities were most culpably imprudent in holding a Public Meeting upon such a subject'.[88] In 1834 a Cambridge printer reminded the local population of the treatment meted out to the poor:

> No help is nigh, a dread and fearful gloom
> Surrounds him with the horrors of his doom.
> A worse than felon's doom! For when his life
> Returns to God! Then, then the bloody knife
> Must to its work – the body that was starved,
> By puppy doctors must be cut and carved:
> Priests of my country! Ye whose Living Head,
> Wept when he saw that Lazarus was dead! –
> Can ye unmov'd with hearts as hard as Burke;
> Behold the scalping knife thus do its work.[89]

As we shall see in the following chapter, the riot was the start of an almost total collapse in the Cambridge University body supply, and the consequences were felt to an even greater extent by the University in Oxford.

In 1835 a riot was sparked in Sheffield by an incident in the Medical School where the caretaker had beaten his wife and the woman had run out of the house screaming of murder. A crowd quickly gathered, believing that an attempt had been made to 'burk' the woman, but the grievances of the crowd had been festering for some time. On attacking the school, the rioters discovered skeletons and dissected bodies. The school was destroyed by the direct action of the crowd on 26 January 1835, although the bodies were later found to have been obtained legally through the Anatomy Act.[90]

Sheffield was the subject of much concern to the Anatomy Inspector in the following years. The threat to the peaceful working of the Act in the city began before the riot in late 1834, when Samuel Roberts, champion of the poor, wrote a pamphlet objecting to the use of the bodies of the poor as a 'dreadful infringement of all humanity and justice'.[91] Roberts's protests continued into the 1840s, and his publications were a thorn in the side of the Anatomy Inspectorate. In a letter to Alfred Austin, poor law commissioner in Manchester, the Anatomy Inspector, John Bacot, wrote:

> I may state to you that we are aware that some persons have been endeavouring to excite the public mind against the Anatomy Act – One individual in particular, who, a few years ago, made a similar attempt has been very active ... we believe, through his instigation that several petitions have, during this session, been presented to the House of Commons against the Anatomy Bill. It is thought very desirable that the public attention should not be roused on the subject of dissection, as thereby prejudices would be excited and more impediments thrown in the way of the study of Anatomy.[92]

Bacot's concern was over questions being asked in Parliament about the rumours of body sales in Sheffield, contained in a handbill signed by Samuel Roberts claiming that 'the body of poor Darwin had been absolutely cut up into quarters and sold for nine shillings a quarter'.[93] The Sheffield and Cambridge riots are notable because they were sparked by the provisions of the Act and led to direct assaults upon anatomy schools.

Conclusion

The government was galvanized into action on anatomy schools after the conviction of medical men for receiving stolen bodies. The later discovery that the ultimate result of a market economy in body supply was murder allowed the introduction of legislation. All classes of society were at risk of bodysnatching, but the Anatomy Act specifically targeted the bodies of the poor. It is, however, difficult to discern specific fears about post-mortem anatomizing in the poor population. There were no direct expressions of anger, but evidence of antipathy is apparent when other examples of social disorder are examined. The introduction to Dorothy Thompson's *The Early Chartists* claims that one stimulus for Chartism was 'the exclusion from citizenship in the Reform Act', but there were other factors, including 'the Anatomy Act and the pursuit of the propertyless beyond the grave'.[94] The Anatomy Act was passed at a time of wider concerns over franchise reform and mortal disease, and much of the furore is therefore hidden from immediate view, concealed within other expressions of social disorder. Examination of Hansard illustrates that the passing of the Anatomy Act was quite literally hidden away, with debates taking place at unsociable hours and in the wake of more pressing legislation.

The poor of Manchester, along with other urban populations, articulated their anger during the cholera riot, when the community was under particular threat – when social mores, notably burial practices, were disturbed. The discovery of 'burking' activity in Manchester also certainly incited the poor population to action. There is, however, little evidence of direct public concern over the Anatomy Act in Oxford, despite the presence of a small yet significant number of poor people. In 1772 the population stood at around 11,000, which included between 1,500 and 3,000 seasonal inhabitants attached to the university. In 1801 the populace was still under 12,000, and although within twenty years it had grown by 50 per cent,[95] early nineteenth-century Oxford remained a moderately sized market town, primarily known for, and dominated by, the university. Despite its romantic image as a market town with 'dreaming spires', Oxford's economy was based on low pay and seasonal work dependent on the weather and the university; indeed, in very bad weather it became 'a starvation town'.[96] The colleges employed large numbers of people engaged in domestic service, but they were closed for half the year, thereby creating sudden periods of widespread unemployment. However, the presence of large numbers of influential clergy in the colleges appears to have given the poor some level of protection from the workhouse.

Oxford was a key centre of charitable giving, and the founders of Oxford charitable organizations went on to found the London-based Charity Organization Society. Oxford later became a shining example in the campaign against outdoor relief. Much of this provision was met by the large number of unoccupied women attached to academics at the university. The threat of ending up in the workhouse in Oxford was small, and the surviving evidence later suggests that even in the event of death in the workhouse, the Guardians went to great lengths to secure decent funerals for paupers. The poor body supply in Oxford under the Anatomy Act and the fluctuating fortunes of the Manchester anatomy schools is the subject of the next chapter.

The terms of the Anatomy Act were extremely vague, allowing for a wide interpretation of the law and access for surgeons to a wide variety of institutions. The ability of the poor to articulate their wishes within the workhouse, asylum and hospital was seriously limited by the secrecy around the legislation, and there was no compulsion to inform the poor about their rights. There was no definition of who could claim a body and what obligation any claimant then had to pay for a burial. The discretionary nature of the Anatomy Act allowed for a variety of actions by poor law authorities, and certainly in the cases of Manchester and Oxford there was actually no great enthusiasm for widespread dissection of pauper bodies. This early recalcitrance on the part of parish officers to adopt the Act and the efforts of central government to encourage them to adopt its provisions is the subject of the next chapter.

4 THE WORKING OF THE ANATOMY ACT IN OXFORD AND MANCHESTER

The previous chapter traced the passage of legislation addressing the issues raised by surgeons and anatomists, outlined the perceived shortage of bodies and the anxiety over criminality, and reviewed the resulting reaction of those most at risk from the provisions of the Anatomy Act. The promises of an increased supply of cadavers were not realized evenly across the anatomy schools. The passing of the Anatomy Act did not lead immediately to the freeing up of large numbers of cadavers despite the concern expressed by the poor. The Act allowed for the use of the unclaimed poor and caused much anxiety within vulnerable groups, but it had to be adopted and enforced and this was certainly not guaranteed. Poor law authorities were often reluctant to give up bodies and preferred to bury workhouse residents.

The perceived shortage of cadavers allowed the eventual dominance of medical education by hospital medical schools supplied by their own mortuaries. The inability of the smaller (and cheaper) schools to compete in access to bodies led ultimately to their demise. The private schools also found it difficult to compete due to the metropolitan bias of the Royal College of Surgeons. Much of this chapter will focus on the decline of independent medical schools in Manchester and the failure of the university medical school in Oxford.

This chapter aims to examine cadaver supply and shortage through an extensive analysis of the Anatomy Inspectorate records, illustrating the importance of the relationship between competing schools and the Anatomy Inspector. The work is of course hampered by the covert nature of anatomy even after the Anatomy Act and the incomplete official record, which deteriorates significantly after 1870. The present research does, however, indicate that Oxford University, despite the presence of the Radcliffe Infirmary, did not adapt to the new surgical demands of the profession but rather continued to concentrate on the creation of gentlemen scholars immersed in the study of natural philosophy. These scholars became the elite physicians concentrated in major metropolitan centres, but they were a group declining in status and influence within the medical hierarchy. Part of Oxford's inability to adjust was based on a lack of cadavers for anatomy education. The Manchester schools differed, going to great lengths to ensure a decent delivery of bodies. Fundamental to this supply was the relationship cultivated by one anatomy teacher, Thomas Turner, with the Inspector of Anatomy. His school became the dominant private school in Manchester and ultimately the foundation for medical studies at Owens College and the Victoria University. Chapter 1 examined the struggle that the private teachers of Manchester and the doctors of the infirmary had with the Royal College of Surgeons to get their courses and institutions recognized, and so it is important to acknowledge that the College was antagonistic towards teaching outside of the metropolitan centres. The Anatomy Office records, however, illustrate that while the by-laws of the Royal College were a key aspect of the fall of the private schools, the Inspector also berated the existence of competing schools and worked with individuals in the regions to reduce the number of anatomy schools and therefore concentrate body supply within one institution.

This chapter makes a detailed study of the correspondence of the Anatomy Inspector with the schools in Manchester and Oxford (and Cambridge, as a contrast), and a complete list of student numbers and cadaver numbers and sources (where they exist) for the years 1832–1900 is compiled within the appendix. Body supply was vital for the success of a school, and despite the various mergers that took place in Manchester over the course of the century, its schools went into a serious decline in student numbers between 1860 and 1873, when Manchester Royal, the largest provincial school, was overtaken by other provincial centres. This work contends that this is certainly partly due to low cadaver numbers as well as the lack of full-time teachers and professors. These disadvantages were not overcome until Manchester Royal was successful in its bid to become part of the ambitious Owens College.

Body Supply and the Decline of Private Medical Schools

While the poor in workhouses paid the ultimate penalty for the Anatomy Act, one major victim was the private medical school, with its cheaper and more accessible medical education. The first Anatomy Inspector, James Somerville,[1] was conscious from the very start that the Act was hugely flawed and would lead ultimately to the failure of the private schools and the elevation of hospital anatomy schools. In one early report, Somerville said that the Act was 'immediately destructive to the usefulness of the private schools, or those not connected with hospitals'.[2] There was no compulsion on the part of parish authorities to give up their dead and no means of controlling the body supply between institutions. In some cases, and certainly in Manchester and Oxford, the workhouses could be extremely reluctant to give up bodies to the anatomists, preferring to bury bodies at public expense. Schools attached to teaching hospitals could override sporadic shortages by relying on post-mortem examinations to demonstrate anatomy to students. There were, however, many governors who demonstrated a profound commitment to the welfare of the poor within their institutions. The Radcliffe Infirmary went to great lengths to attempt to control the level of dissection and post-mortem activity within the hospital.

From the start there was disappointment experienced by some London anatomists at what they saw as the scarcity of bodies for dissection due to the intransigence of the parochial authorities. In one case, that of Spitalfields, Somerville expressed his annoyance that a register of the wishes of workhouse residents was being kept and that they chose burial over dissection:

> Your parish while they adopt the Bill have accompanied its operation with such provisions as effectually to render it nugatory – For while in other Parishes the inmates of the Workhouses are left to be guided by their own feelings the plan adopted by yours of recording their wishes effectually defeats your intentions.[3]

The body supply could only be secured when parish authorities were in favour of the Act and when the poor were not made completely aware of its terms and so encouraged to opt out of the system. Somerville understood that the less the Act was in the public eye, the better. He hoped nothing would happen 'to excite the feelings of the poor against the operation of this enactment', and he called continually for 'great discretion' from the metropolitan anatomists.[4] The supply was affected particularly adversely in London from 1838 during a vociferous campaign in workhouses by the surgeon William Roberts.[5] Fifty years later inspectors were still demanding secrecy in order to protect the body supply:

> Every act of indiscretion on the part of any of the authorities concerned with the supply of subjects for dissection allows an opportunity for the editors of newspapers to indulge their propensity of pandering to the prejudices of the unlearned which invariably arrests or diminishes the supply of subjects.[6]

A scandal brought an almost immediate shortage of bodies. This was recognized at the outset, when the salary for the Inspector of Anatomy was set in 1832 to be paid out of an allocated fund rather than through the normal channel of Parliament. The Home Office records note that 'an annual discussion on this delicate subject is very much to be deprecated and would probably lead to increasing difficulty (great enough already) in procuring bodies for dissection for the schools of anatomy'.[7]

It is tempting to speculate that the gradual growth of coronial post-mortems may have supplied teaching opportunities when bodies were scarce through the provisions of the Anatomy Act. The *Lancet* among others certainly called for increasing the number of coronial post-mortems: 'were we to be asked whether we believe that the utility of the Coroner's inquest would be increased by the institution of the post-mortem examination in all cases of sudden death ... we should emphatically reply yes'.[8] However, the numbers of such post-mortems were small and there was no necessity for them to be conducted by teachers or specialists. Most autopsies were conducted by the local general practitioner, often the doctor who had recently treated the patient. There was much criticism that these doctors did not conduct full post-mortems but simply looked for a cause of death that immediately conformed to their own recent clinical diagnosis. They also yielded to the 'entreaties of relatives and friends not to extend the examination further than was absolutely necessary'.[9] The efficacy of this type of operation in teaching was obviously extremely limited.

Hospital anatomy schools were better placed to take advantage of a competitive system, particularly when there was a shortage of bodies. In the case of Guy's Hospital, preferential admission to the sick poor was granted to parishes that allowed the hospital access to its parish dead, and St Bartholomew's paid high 'fees' to one parish undertaker.[10] Somerville's attempts to institute a fairer system between hospital and private schools based on student numbers were continually thwarted by teachers who were prepared to invent students. Hospitals could of course benefit by deaths within the institution, and as already noted in Chapter 2, the numbers of hospital post-mortems, with or without permission, is impossible to quantify. It is difficult to resist the notion that surgeons would use hospital post-mortems as a teaching tool in addition to its diagnostic role. In 1826 there were eight independent anatomy schools in London[11] and four hospital schools.[12] By 1871 there were no private schools but a further seven hospital schools.[13]

Somerville himself was disappointed with the supply from the start,[14] and he managed to do little to rectify the problem. The supply in London in Somerville's last season of office (1841–2) was 36 per cent lower than it had been in his first.[15] While the supply in most years was no worse than that experienced in the days of the resurrection men, the raised expectations of medical men as a result of government action were not met, and the result was the removal of Somerville from office in 1842. He had failed to make allies in either the London medical establishment centred on the Royal College of Surgeons or among the teachers of the private schools.

Manchester Schools and the Anatomy Inspectorate

Joseph Jordan was the first to give a set of organized anatomy lectures and demonstrations in Manchester from 1812, and his school later became known as the Mount Street School. Thomas Turner began teaching in a more fully organized school at Pine Street in 1824, eventually taking over Jordan's institution. In 1829 Thomas Fawdington (1795–1843),[16] after serving four years as lecturer in pathology at Mount Street, founded the Marsden Street School along with

Thomas Boutflower (1797–1889),[17] which lasted for ten years. This school became uneconomic: in 1839 it had just fourteen students to Pine Street's sixty-five.[18] Arthur Dumville (1813–71)[19] and George Southam (1815–76)[20] started the Chatham Street School in 1850, and this school ran successfully until 1856, when it amalgamated with Pine Street. These mergers will be examined in detail, particularly the takeover of Jordan's school by Turner in 1836. It is apparent that this development was very probably a direct result of the Anatomy Act and sporadic shortages of bodies over the period. Turner's dominance was assisted by his relationship with the office of the Anatomy Inspector.

A survey of Somerville's London correspondence with parish officers 'yields a wide use of name-dropping, influence and manipulation of power, which was quite frequently based on bluff'.[21] This was echoed in the provinces, and the Inspectorate records are full of complaints from outraged and disappointed provincial anatomists. Somerville was concerned about this from the very start of the new office, and the problem followed successive inspectors. In a letter to Edward Wallis in Hull on 2 October 1832, Somerville wrote, 'The difficulties that you apprehend are similar to those experienced in London and in several other places, but I cannot help thinking that by your perseverance you will ultimately succeed in overcoming the prejudices to which you allude'. On the same date he wrote to Mr Sands Cox in Birmingham: 'I regret to hear that you are likely to meet with any opposition more especially from such a source but I trust the governors of the Hospital will be made fully sensible of your claims'.[22]

One of Somerville's immediate tasks was to outline the extent of anatomy instruction available in the provincial towns, listing student numbers and bodies available for the previous session of study.[23] Manchester had two recorded schools, but the return did not include Jordan's school, which failed to submit any figures. Pine Street had sixty-four students dissecting thirty bodies, and Marsden Street had thirty pupils and seventeen bodies.[24] These figures indicate that Manchester was by far the biggest centre for anatomy and dissection outside the metropolitan centre. Immediately after the passing of the Act, the two leading lights of medical teaching in Manchester, at a public dinner to celebrate the new theatre at Pine Street, expressed their optimism for the future and their belief in the importance of Manchester in medical education. One speech-maker

> congratulated the members of the medical profession, in all branches, who were present and he congratulated society, that the time had now arrived when that honourable science might be pursued without those discreditable associations to which it had hitherto been subject ... It was not good on any account, certainly not so as regarded the medical profession, that cases should arise in which people might exclaim in the language of Lear 'handy dandy, which is the justice and which is the thief'. He used the expression because Mr Jordan had spoken of their robbing church-yards.[25]

From the start of the records, there appears to be evidence of a particularly cordial relationship between Somerville and Thomas Turner, and a determination to make a success of the Act. In a letter to Turner early in 1833, Somerville wrote, 'the satisfaction derived from your prospects indeed I may say of your success is not confined to me but is fully participated at the Home Office as well as by Mr Warburton'.[26] Shortly afterwards, John Sharp of Warrington requested a local inspector to aid his search for bodies. Somerville wrote that this was impossible:

> Mr Turner, motivated by the strongest feelings of interest in his profession has, at my request, taken upon himself the duty of correspondent and to him is mainly to be attributed the successful operation of the Bill at Manchester. When a body is available to the schools Mr Turner receives a communication from the master of the workhouse.[27]

In November 1838 Somerville wrote to Mr Fletcher at Birmingham regarding the distribution of bodies among schools, and he referred to Mr Turner in Manchester as 'my friend ... who did not hesitate for one moment to give a fair share of the bodies to each school'.[28]

In 1836 the two Manchester anatomy schools of Turner and Jordan merged, and it seems that the need to consolidate the body supply within one institution is the likely reason. Certainly as early as 1832 the Inspector noted that the large number of private schools in the provinces was not helpful to the workings of the Act:

> The existence of two or more schools in some of the smaller towns where the supply of dead bodies is limited is an evil so self evident that I have endeavoured to impress the advantages of a coalition on the minds of the teachers and I hope successfully in more than one instance.[29]

Given developments, it seems likely that Jordan gave up his school and anatomical museum to Turner in 1834 in return for support from the Turner faction in an election for the post of honorary surgeon at the Manchester Royal Infirmary. On two previous occasions Jordan had been unsuccessful in his bids to join his rival Turner as an infirmary surgeon, but his fortunes were reversed at the end of 1835. He recognized this win at the third attempt as the highlight of his career: 'I have now reached the height of my ambition. I will retire from practice, enjoy mine ease and keep my carriage'.[30] Jordan lectured at Turner's Pine Street School for one year, and his nephew and partner, Edward Stephens, became the permanent lecturer in pathology and morbid anatomy at the school.[31] Joseph Jordan was a keen dissector and apparently continued to conduct post-mortems at the Manchester Union Workhouse for his own private interest after retirement:

> In order to keep pace with surgical progress he used to go to the Manchester Union Workhouse and there perform operations on the dead body. At that time his friend

George Bowring was visiting surgeon and Mr Coveney was the resident medical officer.[32]

There is certainly evidence in the records that dissections continued at Jordan's home in Bridge Street after the amalgamation of the Manchester schools.[33]

The Marsden Street Anatomy School run by Fawdington and Boutflower was the subject of a takeover by Turner in 1839. In the following year Turner gave the address at the opening session of the Pine Street School, stating: 'the cause which has separated the profession and town for years past, in reference to medical education, has ceased to exist. The gentlemen connected with the Marsden Street Institute have resigned their duties'. Turner had successfully consolidated medical teaching within one pre-eminent institution in Manchester. He went on to express his pride at Manchester medical education, indicating his possession of John Hunter's dissecting table: 'it would seem almost as if the glory of London anatomy were travelling northward and that we had arrested it in Manchester'.[34]

Bodies for the Manchester schools came from local workhouses, and there was at first no great concern over the supply from parochial authorities. Certainly, Turner wrote optimistically to the Inspector:

> There exists no difficulty or opposition whatever on the part of the Poor Law Guardians or Public Authorities and the sole reason for our not having had an abundant supply, is literally that there have been comparatively speaking no deaths among the inmates of our workhouses ... never did any public Bill act better than the Anatomy Bill does with us. We have no opposition, no annoyance in any way. We are careful not to offend the public eye, and our removals and interments are conducted with great decency and care.[35]

By 1850 Turner had overcome the competition from Jordan and Fawdington and Boutflower, and he wrote of the future: 'and now that we are in sole possession of the ground wherein to sow the seeds of medical knowledge in this district ... we cannot doubt that the harvest will be abundant'. He was extremely proud of his achievements and claimed the 'largest museum in the provinces, and that there is not a larger one in London, except that of the College of Surgeons', with 10,000 specimens.[36]

The opportunities afforded by teaching, however, soon ensured that he faced competition from a new school run by Dumville and Southam. Dumville received his first body in November 1850, and the Inspector expressed particular concern to the anatomist that the Act would continue to work well in Manchester:

> It will be a cause of much upset to me in every way should anything occur to interrupt its quiet working. Will you bear in mind what I said about the windows of your dissecting room and have them made not to open at the bottom and altogether so arranged that you will not be overlooked by your neighbours.[37]

Within a year the two schools in Manchester were in conflict over the supply of bodies. Both Dumville and Turner were complaining to the Inspector of short-ages, requesting his assistance. In 1851 the Inspector wrote to the governor of Chorlton-upon-Medlock Workhouse requesting an appeal to the Guardians:

> I regret to find that the limited supply is likely to prove detrimental to medical instruction ... When these provisions are faithfully carried out it is scarcely possible to conceive any objection can be urged against a system which both in London and the Provinces has worked so beneficially.[38]

He then communicated with Dumville, 'I much fear that prejudices against the working of the Act might be aired and your present scanty supply even endan-gered'.[39] The Inspector often wrote to the public institutions of Manchester to urge support of the terms of the Act.

Turner and Dumville conducted a jealous feud through the Anatomy Office. Dumville was denied access to cadavers by Turner, who displayed an increasingly high-handed attitude. The former was warned by the Inspector, George Cur-sham,[40] to work with Turner amicably to keep the issue out of the public eye. As discussed in Chapter 3, the Anatomy Act had come to public attention just a few years before in neighbouring Sheffield, with a disturbance whipped up over the dissection of John Darwin from the Sheffield Workhouse. The Inspector wrote to the poor law commissioner, Alfred Austin, in Manchester about his concern over such agitation. There is a reference to 'one individual in particular' who was attempting to present petitions against the Act in Parliament.[41] The Inspector again advised discretion at all times.[42]

The antagonism between the teachers was a threat to the discreet workings of the Act in Manchester, and the Inspector attempted to mediate over the appor-tionment of bodies, which Turner thought his prerogative. Turner was allowed to remain the 'responsible party'[43] but had to be reminded of his duty:

> I have received your return of another body removed from the Manchester Work-house ... and which you have appropriated to the Pine Street School. If Mr Dumville is in want of one should it not have been sent to him as this is the *fourth* body you have had.[44]

The relationship between the surgeons deteriorated over the next few years, and there was an increasing concern over the Manchester supply, which according to Turner had been quite adequate. The Chatham Street School was increasing its student numbers while those of Pine Street remained static. However, cadaver numbers did not balance demand.[45] The Inspector wrote to Dumville: 'I did my best to procure a better supply of subjects when I was at Manchester but you must be quite aware, it is impossible for me or anyone else to make a *certain pro-vision* for this'.[46] Dumville wrote later in the year to complain of the mutilated state of the most recently received body. The Inspector responded with Turner's reason for this: 'Mr Turner informs me all but two out of the eight last received at the school have been in a similar condition'.[47]

Later, in 1852, Inspector Cursham proposed a committee to distribute cadavers, with a representative from each school. Dumville was the representative for his own school, with Mr Smith[48] for the Royal Pine Street School.[49] This solution came too late to repair the relationship between the schools. In October, at the opening of the Chatham Street School, the Inspector was concerned over the public reporting of matters relating to the supply of bodies and wrote to Smith:

> I very much regret that Mr Southam should have been so ill advised as to say what he is reported to have done at the opening of the Chatham Street School. It was the height of imprudence to allude to these matters at all in a report which no doubt was intended to appear in the public papers, but it renders the matter much worse when the statement with reference to their supply is not consistent with the truth. You acted wisely in taking no notice of it ... With my best wishes to Mr Turner.[50]

The *Manchester Guardian* did report on the yearly opening of the Chatham Street School but did not refer to the speech; yet it would seem that Southam was correct in bemoaning the lack of subjects. The Inspector complained in his letter about Southam's comments, but he was concerned over the Chatham Street supply himself. The feud continued through the 1850s. The Inspector had to remind Dumville in December 1852, 'I can only repeat what I stated in my letter of the 20 July last, that I wished the notices of removal be referred to a committee of two teachers'.[51] He did, however, write to Smith the next day, saying that Dumville was angry because 'you virtually ignore his appointment to the anatomical committee by undertaking the whole of the duties yourself'.[52]

It seems likely that the supply of bodies in Manchester was assisted by the amalgamation of Turner's and Jordan's schools. The shortage perceived in the 1850s could simply have been the result of competition with the Chatham Street School. The problem continued, however, even after the 1859 union of the schools into the Royal School of Medicine. In 1856 the Inspector wrote to the chairman of the Salford Board of Guardians, reminding him of his promise to supply bodies once the workhouse had relocated to a quieter district from its previous 'populous neighbourhood':

> By direction of the Home Secretary I have recently made an inspection of the Schools of Anatomy in the provinces and I regret to find that at Manchester the supply of bodies is by no means sufficient for the large number of pupils attending at that important school.[53]

There is no evidence that Salford responded to this query. In January 1857 another appeal was sent: 'I shall be much obliged if you will inform me whether the Board of Guardians are willing to give up their unclaimed bodies in the Salford Union for anatomical investigation.'[54] Despite receiving an assurance of bodies from Salford in February,[55] the Inspector again wrote to the Royal School in December: 'I regret to see you have had such a bad supply of subjects during this session and that at present you have had none from Salford.'[56] The situation was no better in September 1858 – not one body had been released by the Salford Union.

During the 1850s the Salford Union was by no means unusual, and at this time the pattern of body supply seems to resemble that of the London anatomy schools, with complaints about the dearth of cadavers. Shortages were also experienced in the 1850s and 1860s at other provincial schools, notably Birmingham and Bristol. In October 1858 Cursham advised Dumville to follow the practice of the London schools, which employed undertakers to deal with the workhouses:

> The Chorlton Union have a cemetery of their own, close by the Workhouse at Withington and when I called on Mr Edgehill, the Clerk, he alluded to this and seemed to think the facility and little expense with which they could inter bodies was a reason why the Master did not give himself the trouble to send them to the schools. He spoke in a knowing way about this, and I said I had better bear it in mind. Now if you were to employ a Parish undertaker, he would have an interest in doing his best to ascertain when there were any unclaimed bodies.[57]

In November, Cursham, obviously in some desperation, wrote to the Board of Guardians of the Stockport Union and to the governor of the Borough Gaol and New Bailey Prison in Manchester urging these institutions to assist the supply, as well as to Mr Mainwaring, the poor law inspector at Whitehall, requesting his intercession with the local boards. There is no record of the reply, but Cursham did write to Dumville, 'I enclose you the copy of a letter I have received from Mr Mainwaring, it appears to me, we have nothing to expect from him, but opposition.'[58] Further appeals were dispatched to the Prestwich Union and the County Lunatic Asylum. The latter certainly felt unable to assist: 'I am much obliged to the Visitors for their courteous consideration of my request, and regret they felt unable to comply with it, and can only hope that at some future time they may be induced to reconsider their decision.'[59] Even when a favourable reply was received, there was certainly no guarantee that a body would result. Cursham reported that Matthews at Chorlton 'still *promises* well, although I suspect from some cause or other he does not *perform* to the extent of his power.'[60]

The situation for the Manchester School did not improve, and an approach was made to the Ashton-under-Lyne Guardians, although the Anatomy Inspector was unhappy at the distance involved. The Inspector was anxious to avoid a national trade in bodies because transporting bodies increased the likelihood of public awareness of anatomy, as had often been the case at the height of bodysnatching activity before the Act.[61] This reluctance was waived in the cases of Oxford and Cambridge. At the end of 1863, the Inspector was very surprised to note that Manchester's supply for the previous quarter was at an all-time low with two bodies (Liverpool, with half the students, had received nine).[62] The Inspector wrote, 'I never knew such a thing to occur at your school before',[63] and in the following year he started another round of appeals to workhouses.[64] The voluminous correspondence between the Anatomy Office and the poor law authorities demonstrates the power of the local workhouse masters in the working of the Anatomy Act. In a letter to Smith at the Royal School in Manchester, the Inspector wrote about Mr Brokenshire, governor of Chorlton Union workhouse:

> He is much desirous to render any aid in his power and it would be well to keep on good terms with him in case of a scarcity of subjects at the Manchester Workhouse. When Master of the Kensington Workhouse he rendered much valuable service to the metropolitan schools and his resignation of that office has been much felt.[65]

In 1864 Leeds Anatomy School paid the master of the workhouse five pounds per year 'in consideration of his readiness to promote the supply of subjects for dissection', and the Inspector believed the Royal School could benefit from a similar arrangement.[66] Private medical schools had to be prepared to source bodies from a wide hinterland. The Leeds School of Anatomy applied for bodies from Wakefield House of Correction and Asylum, Leeds, Bradford, Halifax and York Workhouses, later Barwick, Holbeck and Hunslett Workhouses, and Leeds Infirmary and House of Recovery, as well as Tadcaster Workhouse in 1875.[67] It seems that Leeds experienced a shortage of bodies in the first few years of operation after the Anatomy Act, but there was some resurgence by 1840. In 1865 the prospectus claimed optimistically that 'the supply of cadavers for dissection continues to be steady and abundant',[68] although the more reliable figures in the Appendix indicate a fluctuating stock.

Much of the evidence for this chapter is taken from the extensive records of the Anatomy Inspectorate, as regrettably most of the poor law records from the Manchester region before the beginning of the century have not survived. There is some evidence to suggest that parishes did make some efforts to bury the unclaimed and unwanted. In August 1834 the Overseers spent seven shillings and six pence 'for the internment of the late female found drowned in the Medlock River'.[69] At the very end of the nineteenth century, when the anatomy records are in fact less detailed, there are a few notes in workhouse burial registers that some unclaimed bodies were being sent for dissection. The burial records for Withington Workhouse indicate several burials at Phillips Park and are annotated '*OC*', suggesting use by Owens College, but the numbers remained small, usually around three or four per month in the early years of the twentieth century.[70] What is more striking, however, is the evidence that the parish continued to bury unclaimed bodies in preference to sending them to the anatomists.[71] Even into the twentieth century the Chorlton Guardians in Manchester were anxious that 'the hospital should not be a practising ground for young doctors'.[72] This is a trend that is very apparent in the records of the Radcliffe Infirmary in Oxford, a theme that will be revisited below.

The returns of student numbers in the anatomy records[73] and the correspondence examined above indicate that the amalgamation of the Chatham Street and Pine Street Schools in the late 1850s did not halt the decline of Manchester anatomy. The Royal School, which under different guises had been the largest provincial medical school from 1800, was overtaken in numbers and reputation by Birmingham around 1860, until the Manchester School re-emerged under the auspices of the Owens College in the later 1870s. The establishment of the college and the role played by the medical wing will be examined in the next chapter.

Oxford University and the Anatomy Inspectorate

In much of this section a comparative approach has been followed with work on Cambridge University Anatomy School. As the only other English university able to confer medical degrees at the time of the Anatomy Act, Cambridge affords a natural point of comparison with Oxford, and the two were often dealt with by the Anatomy Inspector on the same basis. Hurren has found that Cambridge University, in contrast with Oxford University, was energetic in increasing its status as an anatomically focused medical school.[74] The arrival of Michael Foster (1836–1907)[75] and the presence of George Murray Humphrey (1820–96)[76] gave Cambridge the opportunity to establish itself as a leading centre for the study of physiology, a discipline that required a strong grounding in anatomical knowledge. Hurren has demonstrated that the Cambridge University Anatomy Department went to great lengths to ensure that it established a regular supply of cadavers. Professors Acland and Rolleston (1829–81)[77] at Oxford gave little attention to this area and so received very few bodies. Oxford's decline in anatomy was not ultimately arrested until the end of the nineteenth century with the arrival of key personnel, John Burdon-Sanderson (1828–1905)[78] and Arthur Thomson (1858–1935).[79] The latter made an immediate attempt to secure an adequate number of bodies for the re-emerging anatomy school, ultimately with limited success. This impetus is evident in the records of the Anatomy Inspectorate but can also be traced by the records of the new suburban cemeteries of Oxford from 1890.

As small cities, Oxford and Cambridge could never hope to procure the number of bodies available in other anatomical centres; yet the Anatomy Act expressly forbade the transport of bodies from one part of the country to another.

Provincial anatomists were often reminded of this clause by the Inspector, who was always anxious to avoid public scandal:

> I have received yours of the ninth in which you express a desire that a body should be sent to your school from London. By the perusal of the Anatomy Act you will perceive that such a proceeding as the transport of a body from one town to another is not only in opposition to its spirit but directly to its provisions since the burials cannot take place where the individual died and few if any of the Parish Officers will feel disposed to allow the transit of bodies beyond their reach.[80]

In October 1833 the Home Office responded in the strongest terms to requests from Edinburgh University for London bodies:

> Lord Melborne has given this suggestion the fullest consideration and his Lordship has desired one to express to you, in the strongest manner, his decided objection to this mode of obtaining bodies for the schools at Edinburgh, and to inform you, that if any attempts are made to resort to this plan of obtaining bodies the utmost vigilance of the Police will be exerted to detect the person concerned in carrying it on – and to enforce any penalties the existing Law would authorize.[81]

The Home Office expressed concern when Oxford requested bodies from London, as it was worried about 'the risk of excitement from such a course, [which] is far greater than from making use of the bodies in the Town where the lectures on anatomy are delivered'.[82] An exception to this rule was made almost immediately for Cambridge University, evidenced in documents marked 'secret and confidential'. Cambridge had been the site of a recent riot against the Act ('the attempt to make the Act efficient at Cambridge was attended with consequences so alarming that it has not been judged expedient since to repeat the experiment'[83]). Somerville requested that the Home Secretary allow the two universities a small supply from the floating hulks at Woolwich. Cambridge University was allowed two hulk bodies but the request from Oxford was declined, although Oxford University had received one previously from London under the direction of Lord John Russell.[84] In the same communication Somerville expressed his annoyance at a request from Cambridge University for four bodies each session, as the bodies of the convicts were highly prized by anatomists (in preference to the elderly poor, which made up most of the workhouse supply).[85] He noted that the metropolitan provision was shaky and that the anatomists there would be most unhappy not to share this valuable source, in addition to the claims of Oxford University. Cambridge University had complained that the one or two bodies per year allowed from the hulks was enough for a public lecture, resembling a demonstration, but at least four were required for students to undertake their own dissections.[86] In 1835 the anatomy course was suspended for the year.

Bodies from the hulks were scarce (particularly in mild weather), expensive to transport and often subject to post-mortem examination by order of the coroner and so of less value to anatomists. Cambridge University anatomists experienced difficulties with bodies that had already been opened because the local medical man had conducted a post-mortem examination. The university professor was not keen to accept such bodies. The Inspector wrote to John Williams at the Portsmouth hulks:

> I can easily understand that occasions may arise, not infrequently, for post-mortem examination, and that you naturally avail yourself of such opportunities as your position affords for professional improvement. I trust however, that this may not be found incompatible with still preserving to the schools a valuable addition to the supply.[87]

The level of post-mortem examination also appears to have been a problem for the metropolitan schools, with medical officers at the London workhouses undertaking autopsies to further their own education, thereby denying the bodies to anatomy schools.[88] The desire by individual medical men to undertake post-mortem examinations whenever they could was understandable after 1832. One result of the Anatomy Act was to ensure that dissection was only undertaken by licensed anatomists within recognized institutions. The Anatomy Inspectorate records contain much correspondence warning individuals not connected to the schools that the days of simply paying for a body from the resurrection men were over, and that they were unlikely to be able to secure any sort of supply outside of a bona fide anatomy school.[89] Medical men had recognized this as a problem for continuing education from the inception of the first Bill in 1829. One writer to the *Lancet* was horrified to learn that

> dissections can be legally conducted *only* in towns where there are schools conferring degrees in anatomy, or in which there is a hospital containing fifty beds; thus *utterly precluding nine-tenths* of the medical men throughout the country, from keeping up an intimate knowledge of anatomy.[90]

Oxford's supply of bodies appears from the records of the Anatomy Inspectorate to be almost non-existent in the aftermath of the Anatomy Act.[91] The university rarely appears in the list of licensed anatomy schools receiving bodies, yet its rival Cambridge is usually listed. In a letter to Cambridge University, the Inspector requested that Professor Clark (1788–1869)[92] 'defer the practical illustrations of your lectures to as late a period as is consistent with your circumstances as our supply is as yet very scanty, and more particularly from the hulks'.[93] There are sporadic requests over several years from Dr Kidd, Oxford professor of medicine, for a single body, and these were usually granted. This was certainly the case by November 1841, when Somerville wrote to Kidd:

> The directions given to me by Sir James Graham leave nothing to be desired but the opportunity, the mortality at the Hulks has been remarkably small. But you may depend upon my attending to your interests with the least possible delay. If I can get

our affairs on a proper footing it would be a source of great satisfaction for me to be able to accept of your kindness when I visit the Anatomical School at Oxford.[94]

Regrettably for Kidd (and also for Clark at Cambridge), the hulks provided little dissection material in reality, despite the assurances given. The promised body for Oxford had not materialized a month later: 'The want of the means has been the only cause of the delay in my complying with your request – and the orders of the Home Office. The mortality at the Hulks has been as nothing'.[95] Somerville wrote again to regret that a body was unlikely to be available before February or March.[96] There are no further references to Oxford in either the metropolitan or provincial anatomy records, indicating a largely moribund anatomy school.

Cambridge University experienced increasing difficulties with the bodies from the hulks and ultimately of course the complete loss of this as a source of cadavers. By the 1850s the new Inspector was urging the university to develop its links with Addenbrookes Hospital.[97] All Anatomy Inspectors expressed their great concern over the transport of bodies due to the need for secrecy. Packing bodies in cases and sending them long distances risked public scandal, as had occurred on many occasions in the era of bodysnatching. The Act only worked efficiently while its provisions were hidden. Alcock Rutherford, a Metropolitan Inspector, wrote, 'I fear it is very uncertain when I may be enabled with safety or prudence to send you a subject from the metropolitan supply', and he suggested that Cambridge request help from the Provincial Inspector, John Bacot.[98]

The shortage of cadavers experienced by many institutions in the 1850s was also felt by Cambridge University. In a letter to Humphrey, the Inspector regretted 'the insufficient supply of subjects for dissection at that place ... Viscount Palmerston has requested that I would communicate with you'.[99] In the following month Inspector Cursham offered to write to the relevant institutions on Humphrey's behalf, much as he had done for Manchester.[100] Cambridge University finally established a somewhat scanty supply from one workhouse and Addenbrookes Hospital.[101] Humphrey continued to write to the Inspector for assistance. Once the supply from the hulks was curtailed, the Inspector felt less inclined to allow the transportation of bodies from London.

> You are, I believe aware that no bodies are now obtained from the hulks. There would be risk in sending a body by rail lest the contents of the package should be discovered and if such were to be the case a great hubbub would doubtless be raised and the supply to the London schools in all probability most materially damaged.[102]

The Inspector voiced his greatest fear that relatives calling at the relevant workhouse would then discover that the body had been sent to Cambridge University. There had been a scandal when this occurred between the Wolverhampton Workhouse and Birmingham Anatomy School. The Inspector had to write again in almost exactly the same terms two years later after yet another request for bodies to be sent from London.[103]

Oxford University drops out of the Anatomy Inspectorate records completely between 1844 and 1864.[104] There are no letters to Kidd or his successor, Henry Acland, nor are there any student or body returns for this period, suggesting that human dissection ceased completely at Oxford. The records at Christ Church (the Oxford College that housed the university's anatomy school) suggest that there was some expenditure on wax models by the school, and a request for payment for anatomical specimens was refused until there was proof that two bodies had been received and dissected as demanded by the terms of the Lee bequest.[105] The Board of Governors of the Radcliffe Infirmary was at pains to make clear to the clinicians that 'it forbids the dissection of any Patient in the Infirmary for the sake of mere anatomical demonstration'.[106] Post-mortems were allowed, but only with the permission of the relatives, and clinicians were warned against opening bodies for the 'mere purpose of general demonstration'.[107]

There is finally a letter from the Anatomy Inspector in 1861 in reply to an application from Dr Rolleston at Oxford University for a licence to practise anatomy.[108] Three years later the Inspector sent to Rolleston documentation relating to four bodies received at Oxford Anatomy School, and there was no mention of the source.[109] In 1865 the Inspector offered to write to the relevant poor law unions on Rolleston's behalf.[110] A request from Rolleston for London bodies was refused, but a suggestion was made to approach neighbouring unions and the local asylum, as Humphrey at Cambridge had done with some limited success.[111] The Inspector advised Rolleston at Oxford to approach workhouses directly through the medical officer and master, as 'guardians are too often strange mortals to deal with in such delicate subjects'.[112]

It seems that towards the end of the nineteenth century Oxford University managed to establish a small but regular supply of bodies. The out-letter books of the Anatomy Inspectorate suggest that these did not always come from the workhouses but also from the Radcliffe Infirmary, which appears to have reversed its earlier antipathy towards dissection.[113] The Weekly Board of the Radcliffe Infirmary reported in 1886:

> It was resolved that in the event of a patient without friends and without parish settlement dying, the body should be given to the University School of Anatomy, care being taken that it should be moved with all due respect at the cost of the School and receive burial as directed by the Anatomy Act.[114]

This reversal was, however, limited in reality, and there is much evidence that the Radcliffe Infirmary went to great lengths to find claimants for poor cadavers and in many cases buried bodies at the infirmary's own expense rather than send them to the anatomy school. It does not, in other words, appear to have sent bodies to the school unless all other avenues were closed. In August 1899 the house physician requested that the body of infant Albert Nicholls, who had died after his mother's death in the infirmary, be sent to the anatomy school. Mr Nicholls had already refused the body, claiming that Albert had been conceived while he had been in prison. The officers of the infirmary went to great lengths in voluminous correspondence to find another claimant, and they finally ascertained the view of the child's grandparents before acceding to the appeal.[115]

In the many cases of paupers with friends or relatives unable to bury loved ones, the infirmary spent the money on the funeral and then attempted to claim it back from a relevant poor law union, with much resulting argument (and therefore documentary evidence) and often little success.[116] As just one of many examples, in 1896 the infirmary attempted to claim burial expenses from Headington and Thame Unions for a Mrs Hale, 'whose late husband was unable to bury her remains for want of means'.[117] The case was the subject of protracted correspondence over two months. Apart from Albert Nicholls, there is only one other documented instance of a body going to the anatomy school in a complete survey of Radcliffe Infirmary records up to 1904. The second case concerned a traveling showman who was taken ill in Oxford and died suddenly in the infirmary:

> It appearing that the deceased had no known friends and no known parish settlement, it was moved by Dr Brooks and seconded by Mr Symonds and carried unanimously that the body should be handed over to the University School of Anatomy pursuant to the order of the Committee.[118]

Oxford Anatomy School was possibly successful in receiving bodies from the Oxford Union at this time (the records have not survived), but efforts to expand the supply by Professor Rolleston were fraught with difficulty. At a specially convened meeting to consider a letter from Rolleston, the Board of Guardians of neighbouring Headington Union 'resolved unanimously that no unclaimed bodies be allowed to be removed from the Workhouse for the purposes of dissection'.[119] Abingdon Union also refused Rolleston's approach in 1879.[120] Despite the official attitude of Guardians, bodies may of course have been received in private arrangements with the masters of workhouses. The lack of dissection evidence from the Christ Church records supports the contention, however, that practical anatomy ceased at the university for much of the nineteenth century. The evidence from the quarterly returns of bodies dissected sent to the Anatomy Inspectorate demonstrates the occasional body to Oxford from 1834 to 1844, one in 1865 and no further bodies up to 1871 when these records end.[121]

There was a new impetus in 1885, when Arthur Thomson was appointed to the new post of lecturer in human anatomy at Oxford University (hitherto any anatomical lectures were undertaken by the professor of comparative anatomy in zoology) and promised a new anatomy building, which finally opened in 1893.

However, Oxford was a small town dominated by a clerical elite seemingly disposed towards the respectable burial of the poor. The university anatomy school therefore suffered from the same problems outlined by Alexander Macalister (1844–1919), professor of anatomy at Cambridge: 'We have very many difficulties in carrying on a School of Anatomy in a town with a small population in a thinly peopled centre'.[122]

Gradually Cambridge University had increased its supply by bringing bodies from distant sources, a solution that had been frowned upon in the early years of the Anatomy Act. Macalister had been keen to extend his remit further and requested details of how far the metropolitan area of supply extended. He wished to make an appeal to West Ham, Stratford and Greenwich: 'I am sorry to say that the larger East Anglian towns, Norwich, Ipswich and Colchester have a sentimental objection to send us any bodies'.[123] This was exactly Rolleston's experience with the neighbouring Oxfordshire towns. By the end of the nineteenth century the anatomists at Oxford were attempting to follow the methods used previously by Humphrey and Macalister. In 1889 a letter was sent to local Boards of Guardians from J. Bellamy, vice-chancellor, H. G. Liddell, dean of Christ Church, and H. W. Acland, Regius Professor of Medicine, declaring the importance of anatomy for all classes and promising respect for death customs:

> A practical knowledge of the structure of the human body is absolutely essential to the medical man, for without that knowledge it would be impossible to carry on, for the general good, those ministrations to the sick and suffering which form the daily routine of his work. Such knowledge can only be acquired by the examination of the dead ... Rich and poor alike reap the benefit of that skill which such a knowledge can alone bestow.[124]

An influential student guide to medical studies in 1885 noted that Cambridge offered good opportunities for the study of anatomy: 'The opportunities are unsurpassed. But at Oxford the study of human anatomy is prosecuted under difficulties'.[125]

By January 1907 Cambridge University was receiving bodies from workhouses in Luton, Hull, Doncaster, Mildenhall, Bedford, Brighton, Cambridge, Biggleswade, the Three Counties Asylum and Colney Hatch Asylum. The university had been refused by Norwich, Northampton, Leicester, Ipswich, Nottingham, Derby, Portsmouth and Southampton Unions. (Three other Boards of Guardians, including Colchester and Rochester, had agreed to send bodies, but the requests were ultimately refused by the masters of the workhouses.) In 1905 Cambridge also received twelve or thirteen bodies from Manchester[126] despite their complaints over the cost of transport, which were around ten pounds per body.[127] Even with these huge efforts over a very large geographical area, Cambridge was hardly a centre for anatomy and dissection; by 1912 209 medical students were dissecting a mere thirty-one bodies. Manchester was more successful by this period, with 128 students and forty-three bodies supplied by just two workhouses, Manchester and Withington. Oxford University, by contrast, was doing rather well with fifty-two students and sixteen bodies from Leicester, Reading and Oxford Workhouses and the Radcliffe Infirmary. Oxford, alongside all other medical schools, still felt the need to complain to the Anatomy Inspector about supplies even when the situation was obviously fairly reasonable. At a conference on anatomical supply held at the Home Office in 1913, there were complaints from the schools in London, Cambridge and Oxford:

> Manchester seemed to have all they required; everybody else complained that they have no bodies ... the Master of the Workhouse in Manchester is very enthusiastic and takes care that every unclaimed body went to the school. It was peculiar that many of the subjects were Roman Catholics.[128]

This would suggest that supply in anatomy schools could be as a result of the whim of individual workhouse masters. Macalister reported that although he had sent a general letter of appeal to local Boards of Guardians in 1884, 'Guardians refused to see him when he asked for an interview. At Norwich he was practically insulted'.[129]

The *British Medical Journal* reported on the development of the anatomy department at Oxford in 1906. Thomson had become extraordinary professor of human anatomy in 1893, with an average of fifty students per term.

> One serious drawback, however, is the want of an adequate supply of material. The number of unclaimed bodies in Oxford itself is extremely limited, and Guardians in surrounding districts do not show any particular readiness to further the cause of anatomical education; in some cases, indeed, they place difficulties in the way.

The article called for an amendment of the Anatomy Act 'taking the disposal of the unclaimed bodies of persons who die in workhouses out of the hands of Guardians'.[130] It is possible to observe the supply of bodies to the Oxford Anatomy School from the 1890s until 1914 by examining the burial registers for the new suburban cemeteries of Rose Hill, Wolvercote and Botley.[131] The most useful register is that for Botley, as the notation 'museum' has been made against a substantial number of entries; it seems almost certain (given the addresses of the individuals) that this refers to the Anatomy School, located by this time in the Oxford Natural History Museum. This register therefore gives body numbers for all the Oxford sources. The other two registers contain fewer cases, and there is no sure way of ascertaining dissection cases from Oxford. All that can be gleaned is a small number of bodies from outside Oxford, mainly Reading.[132] Manchester supplied a number of bodies buried at Wolvercote and Botley, but only for the years 1907 and 1908. The other chief source was Leicester Workhouse, with bodies buried in Botley cemetery. This was an important location for the anatomy school, as the *Hospital* reported in 1910 that twenty-one bodies had been sent to Oxford in three years:

> At a recent meeting of the Leicester Guardians a resolution was moved to the effect that no more dead bodies should be sent to the Anatomical Society at Oxford University. The mover stated that in his opinion poor people never benefited by medical science, but were exploited while they were alive and when they were dead. It was the bodies of the rich that should be handed over for anatomical research, for it was the rich who gained by such knowledge. The seconder, a lady, said they all knew the importance of anatomical experiments, but as a Guardian she objected to sending the bodies of those who had been under their care to Oxford.[133]

The resolution was lost by twenty-four to thirteen votes, and Leicester Workhouse continued to send bodies to Oxford University.

The records of the municipal burial companies held at the Oxford City Archives indicate that by 1915 Oxford Anatomy School was receiving around twelve bodies per year. Thomson complained about the private burial companies:

> The remains are brought from towns at a distance where the population is much larger than in Oxford. For the burial of these I am charged at present double the rate that I would have to pay had they been Oxford residents.[134]

Thomson also protested over the rate at which bodies were transported to Oxford from Reading and Leicester by the Great Western Railway, at one shilling per mile, but the railway refused to reduce the rate.[135] The anatomy school at Oxford, along with all other medical schools, benefited from the development of formaldehyde as a preserving agent from around 1893, and the university was allowed to keep bodies for up to two years from 1916, but the late start experienced by Oxford University in anatomical education held it back as a clinical school in the nineteenth and early twentieth centuries. Medical students at Oxford, even after the developments outlined above, undertook their final clinical years at London medical schools.

Conclusion

Medical education in the nineteenth century was rooted in the study of anatomy, which gave rise to an enthusiasm for dissection by medical students. In order to survive, private medical schools had to be prepared to search beyond the locality for bodies, and few could rely on a local supply. In the early years after the Anatomy Act the future of the medical faculty at Cambridge University was 'in serious doubt', thanks solely to the poor supply of bodies.[136] The arrival of George Murray Humphrey in 1842 and his assiduous efforts to procure bodies ensured the eventual flourishing of the medical school.

Oxford anatomists never managed to secure a local supply, and Thomson's efforts to modernize the Oxford anatomy school came very much later than other institutions. Henry Acland, professor of medicine at Oxford University during the middle of the nineteenth century (a key period for the acceptance of anatomy in medical education), regarded dissection as unsuitable for undergraduates. His successor, George Rolleston, was equally ambivalent, although as noted Rolleston made some attempts to source bodies. Cadaver supply was always going to be problematic in a small city like Oxford, but such difficulties were largely overcome in Cambridge. The anatomists at Cambridge University worked assiduously to secure bodies from a wide area and also developed a key relationship with the neighbouring hospital. The same cannot be said for Oxford and the Radcliffe Infirmary (where again Acland was a key personality in his role as honorary surgeon). Once the scanty hulk supply dried up, there is no evidence of bodies from any institution finding their way to Oxford anatomy school until the 1860s, when the Infirmary reversed its earlier antipathy to a very limited extent. A few bodies then became available from Oxford, Leicester and Reading Workhouses.

The continuing hostility of the local population to dissection in both Oxford and Manchester is apparent, with both centres having difficulty with a local supply after 1832. The Royal School of Medicine and Surgery in Manchester did not manage to arrest its decline in student numbers until the school became a faculty of Owens College in 1872, when it once again became the pre-eminent provincial medical school, with an increased number of students.

To protect its own metropolitan teachers, the Royal College of Surgeons moved against provincial teaching with petty by-laws. The evidence of the Anatomy Inspectorate illustrates that body supply was a factor in the provision of anatomical training. Manchester's early success as a centre for medical education was based on its history as a vibrant centre of bodysnatching before the Anatomy Act. While individuals such as Thomas Turner attempted to obtain a reasonable legal supply and ensured the good offices of the Anatomy Inspector in local disputes, the body supply became a disappointment for some time. Manchester's decline in student numbers in the period of the 1850s can be linked to an inadequate supply of bodies due to the intransigence of the parochial authorities in aiding anatomical education. The records for the years after 1870 are patchy in the anatomy archives, but Manchester was once again the leading provincial medical school through Owens College from the end of the nineteenth century, and at times it even became an exporter of bodies to other schools (notably Cambridge and Oxford universities).

The Anatomy Act was a key factor in the decline of the independent anatomy schools of London. The evidence from Manchester and Oxford, largely from the Anatomy Inspectorate records, would at least partially support this contention. Even the metropolis could not support small competing private schools, and hospital medical schools were best placed to overcome local shortages with a guaranteed supply of bodies. Anatomy had established itself as the pre-eminent medical discipline in the education of doctors in the nineteenth century. Its role in the later development of medical education nationally and locally is the subject of the final chapter.

5 MEDICAL EDUCATION IN OXFORD AND MANCHESTER AFTER THE ANATOMY ACT

The previous chapter dealt largely with the erratic supply of bodies to the medical schools of Manchester and Oxford in the wake of the Anatomy Act. We now turn to the resulting responses of Oxford and Manchester in the provision of anatomically focused medical education demanded by the General Medical Council in the second half of the nineteenth century. This chapter considers firstly the enduring dominance of anatomy in the medical curriculum (perhaps to the detriment of other specialties such as physiology) and therefore the continuing dependence on large numbers of bodies, by examining the development of Oxford and Manchester medical schools in the latter half of the nineteenth century. The previous chapter provided some evidence to support the claim that private anatomy schools lost out to hospital schools in the metropolis due to the latter's better access to bodies for dissection, the lynchpin of surgery. That conclusion is certainly accurate; private schools did disappear, not only in London but also elsewhere, to be replaced by medical schools attached to hospitals. However, as this chapter aims to demonstrate, it is necessary to examine the wider development of medical education in the nineteenth century, particularly outside the metropolis.

The records at Oxford University, which are in good condition for this later period, demonstrate that the medical staff of the university felt unable to compete with metropolitan and provincial medical schools and so promoted their own medical department as an elite preparatory school for metropolitan high-fliers. The Manchester archives are less well preserved and stored, and so it is difficult to chart its development in the same detail. It does seem, however, that the medical school saw an important opportunity to elevate its qualification by linking formally with Owens College, with its strong reputation for science teaching.

The present chapter examines the growing dominance of the teaching hospital in delivering medical education in the second half of the nineteenth century. The hospital medical school was a more efficient way of providing medical education, as theory could be immediately linked to practice at the bedside (or in the mortuary). Much of this evidence can be found in the *British Medical Jour-*

nal. Additionally, doctors were often keen to promote teaching within their own hospitals, as it assisted claims to professional status against the control of lay governors. The present chapter offers evidence that doctors attempted to continue the development of the more limited post-mortem examination as a teaching tool in the absence of bodies for dissection. However, many doctors still struggled to secure permission for post-mortem examinations in voluntary hospitals.

Dominance of Anatomy in the Medical Curriculum

As we saw in Chapter 1, early nineteenth-century medical education in England was dominated by the study of normal anatomy and practical dissection in contrast to continental Europe, where attention was on morbid anatomy that used the post-mortem 'to detect some marked difference, by which the disease may be distinguished in the living body'.[1] Critics were concerned that this English focus on minute dissection of parts of the normal human body was detrimental to a full 'knowledge of the *living* body' which was the focus of the new discipline of physiology.[2] By the late nineteenth century there was increasing concern that England was falling behind Europe in developing medical science, notably in the field of physiology. In 1872 John Burdon-Sanderson told the British Association section on anatomy and physiology that 'we English physiologists ... must admit with regret that we have had very little to do with the unprecedented development of our science during the last two decades'.[3] Michael Foster agreed: 'the overweening importance still attached to anatomy in our medical schools, to the utter depression of physiology, is a remnant of conservatism from which a liberal education ought to free itself'.[4]

The *British Medical Journal* noted the enduring legacy of anatomy: 'the more recently developed science of physiology is more and more vindicating its place as the scientific basis of that part of medical science which is not purely empirical'.[5] When compared to Europe, there was a relative failure of English physiology: 'continental physiologists were freeing their discipline from its subservience to anatomy'.[6] The reasons for the stagnancy of English physiology and other experimental sciences include much anti-vivisection sentiment and the anatomical bias of English medical education. More importantly, however, the science suffered at the hands of the two traditional English universities. The stagnation only ended with the arrival of Michael Foster at Cambridge. The late elevation of physiology added to Cambridge University's reputation as a medical school, with the largest number of entrants after St Bartholomew's in 1883. The body supply was still important, and Cambridge had around one hundred students dissecting at this time. Oxford University was a latecomer to the discipline of physiology, and as we have seen in the previous chapter, it did not engage with the growth of anatomy in the medical curriculum.

Medical Education and Anatomy at Oxford University

Oxford University's failure to keep pace with changes in medical education was based partly on an inability to procure cadavers for the dominant fields of study. Cambridge University made attempts to overcome this problem, but it also managed to carve out a reputation as the most advanced medical school in Britain by the 1870s, based on the elevation of the practical arm of anatomy, physiology. In contrast, there was a continuing focus in Oxford on an extensive knowledge of music, literature, classical texts, art and natural philosophy. Graduate physicians from Oxford and Cambridge believed that they benefited from a scholarly medical training and had acquired the moral character required to be trustworthy and wise advisers. This impression had significantly diminished as marketplace medicine developed. Despite a late attempt in the 1880s to extend the Oxford Medical School based on the elevation of physiology through the appointment of John Burdon-Sanderson as professor and his efforts to increase students and resources, the school has been considered to be a failure.

Henry Acland has been celebrated in Oxford as a modernizing influence within medical education, and he certainly did much to regulate studies and examinations at the university. Raising the standards for arts students, however, ensured that it was more difficult for students to pass on to medical degrees, and so, while standards were higher, there were fewer attracted to the study of medicine and science. Acland believed himself to be a reformer and a supporter of 'scientific medicine', yet he would not give up his demands that medical students at Oxford complete the arts degree before undertaking medical studies, making Oxford medical education expensive and time-consuming at eight years' duration. An examination of Acland's career provides the opportunity to trace Oxford medical education in an era dominated firstly by the study of anatomy and later by the study of physiology. The particular institutional and individual characteristics of Oxford University are the focus of this section.

After clinical training at St George's and Edinburgh, Acland became Lee's Reader in Anatomy at Oxford University and fellow of All Souls College in 1845, honorary physician to the Radcliffe Infirmary two years later, and Regius and Clinical Professor of Medicine in 1857. His biographer claimed that Acland 'never wavered in his single-minded desire to advance scientific teaching in the University of Oxford, and to serve the cause of medical education in its truest sense'.[7] His central reforming ideas are summarized in a pamphlet produced early in his career that illustrated his rather limited view of Oxford as a medical school:

> If an additional school were wanted, I do not think Oxford the best place for such school. Oxford is a county town of no large size, so that the hospital cases are far more limited in number than in the metropolis of this or other countries; a large field for clinical observation is absolutely necessary for a good Medical School.[8]

Acland was instrumental in the reform of the examination system for medical students at Oxford, but the course could never be more than an introductory study of medicine in preparation for professional training. He held 'long-cherished views on the necessity of a liberal education for those about to be entered on the physic line'.[9] In 1852 he wrote that 'the University should keep strictly to her line of teaching *fundamental* sciences and giving Degrees in *Arts*'.[10]

Acland is an example of the nineteenth-century medical man who espoused the cause of scientific medicine without any analysis or understanding of the term. Science could be used as a convenient rallying cry for professional status by medics who disliked the growth of expensive laboratory medicine and a professional ethic that took no account of the general liberal, classical education associated with genteel status. For medical men like Acland, their expertise in scientific medicine was based on empirical observation and character over experiment and expert training. His legacy, the Natural History Museum in Oxford, is testament to his belief in the unity of knowledge and his dislike of over-specialization.

Chapter 2 demonstrated that the anatomy schools of Manchester benefited greatly from the private anatomical collections of men such as Jordan, Turner and especially Fawdington. The archives at Christ Church College suggest that the anatomical collection that was later placed in Acland's new museum building was extremely limited in its human collections but quite rich in animal exhibits. The lack of human specimens supports the contention that 'where the scope of human collections was limited, comparative anatomy flourished, often to an unusual extent'.[11]

The study of human anatomy at Oxford continued its inexorable decline under the guidance of Acland (who had actually been horrified by his first exposure to a dissection at St George's) and George Rolleston, despite the latter's own research interest in the study of human skeletal remains. In 1869 John Barclay-Thompson became Lee's Reader in Anatomy, but there is no evidence that he dissected any human bodies during his career. For over thirty years he offered a course of lectures on 'the skeleton and teeth of lothyopsida and sauropsida with the leading facts of their distribution in space and time'.[12] Acland as Lee's Reader readily dispensed with human dissections, believing them to be unsuitable for his amateur audiences. By the 1860s Acland's Oxford reputation was established; he became honorary physician to the Prince of Wales in 1863 and ended his career as president of the General Medical Council (1874–87). Yet later in the century there was an acknowledgment that he had not recognized the emerging force of surgery and the importance of establishing Oxford as a premier medical school, and thus the Oxford Medical School continued its decline. In 1868, during a tribute to the science of Morgagni and Hunter, Acland 'cautioned that the exigencies of medical practice and the emergencies daily encountered by the physician precluded him from reliance on the ... uncertainties of scientific medicine'.[13]

In 1878 a controversial debate emerged in the letters page of the *British Medical Journal* under the heading of 'A Lost Medical School' and included a personal attack on Acland.[14] Later in the same year, the professor of zoology at University College London, Edwin Ray Lankester (1847–1929),[15] fellow of Exeter College and later professor at Oxford, added to the criticism by denying the distinction between preliminary and professional studies and outlining the importance of connecting theory and practice. He disapproved of Acland's obsession over the building of the University Museum, which he dismissed as 'a sort of Gothic palace'.[16] He wrote to the *British Medical Journal*, claiming somewhat ambitiously that the Radcliffe Infirmary was 'one of the best fields for clinical instruction in the kingdom'.[17] Lankester wrote to his future colleague John Burdon-Sanderson at University College, complaining of 'the annoyance of delay and opposition at Oxford and the immense dead-weight of inertia which has to be pushed against there'.[18] Lankester was supported by the editor of the *British Medical Journal*, who was highly critical of Acland holding three separate professorships at Oxford: Regius Professor of Medicine, Aldrichian Professor of Medicine and Lichfield Medical Professor.

> Here we have a Regius Professor of Medicine and a Clinical Professor of Medicine, who during the whole term of his office, extending over nearly twenty years, has never, as far as we can find, given either a course of lectures on medicine or a course of clinical instruction in medicine; whose notices to students that he would meet and confer with them, with the view of making arrangements for such courses, have never resulted in anything but vacuous emptiness.[19]

Lankester, a forceful character, was keen to promote English physiology, which he believed was vital to the study of medicine, in an acrimonious dispute in the pages of the *British Medical Journal*. He wrote that the professor of physiology at Oxford (Rolleston) 'does not occupy himself with physiology'.[20] He expressed his frustration that physiology was not understood by the public or government, and that Oxford had done little to help the situation, partly by its insistence on artificially dividing medical education into a theoretical strand and a practical strand. The article reiterated Lankester's belief in the efficacy of the Radcliffe Infirmary as a clinical school and held that the population of Oxford was similar to those of German cities with thriving medical schools, such as Jena and Heidelberg.

A spirited debate emerged within Hebdomadal Council (the governing body of the university) through the 1870s and 1880s, with Acland attempting to limit Oxford's role within clinical medicine. Acland had never accepted the compromise that Cambridge managed, of adapting scientific teaching within the arts degree to the needs of the preclinical medical students. He was also determined to maintain the eight years required for the Oxford Bachelor of Medicine degree despite its obvious unsuitability to the demands of the new General Medical

Council, which required qualifications in physic and surgery. He wished to keep the literary emphasis of the degree and ignore the demands of professional examination. He stated in a memo of 1874 to the medical committee of Hebdomadal Council that 'our graduates are to hold an honourable place as men of general culture and professional attainment'.[21]

Acland took much criticism in the pages of the *British Medical Journal* in the years following the 'lost medical school' debate. In 1879 the journal printed a notice from the *Oxford University Gazette* reporting that Professor Acland 'will be happy to receive members of the University, who may desire information or help in respect of medical study ... on all Mondays in February at noon'. The notice came from the Mathematics and Physical Science Department, as there was no medical faculty. The *British Medical Journal* responded:

> The notion of the Regius Professor of Medicine beginning in the middle of February to bestir himself (nominally) to confer with medical students on their studies, is too intensely ludicrous to be intended for any other than lay understanding. This is the stock notice by which the few officials who read the *University Gazette* have for many years been deluded into the idea that the Regius Professor really does something, and that there really is somewhere in Oxford a medical student of the University, and somewhere in Oxford something which represents a medical school; which, however, unhappily there is not.[22]

The article went on to praise Professor Humphrey at the Cambridge University Anatomy Department, with sixty students dissecting bodies.

For most of the period under examination, Oxford University continued to regard itself as a centre for the academic training of physicians, and the leaders of the medical school failed to foresee the growing importance of morbid anatomy and the subsequent rise of surgery as the dominant therapy. Acland was an influential member of a declining yet tenacious medical elite that emphasized the values of classical and general education and elevated the development of character over experience and clinical excellence. The changing power relations between the branches of medicine hurt the university severely. This was perhaps inevitable given its location in a small provincial city within reasonable distance of the metropolis. Although the city possessed a large and popular infirmary, there was no tradition of surgical training to push forward the demand for better anatomical education. The limited needs of the pure physician were probably met by the Anatomy School, and given the relative wealth of Oxford students, there was no barrier to further studies in London, Edinburgh or Europe. John Seymour Sharkey supported Acland's position regarding Oxford, noting the proximity of London and that 'pathology would fare badly in a place where the mortality would be so low and autopsies so few'.[23]

Acland's critics testified that his attitude to anatomy and dissection as well as his disregard for rising specialties such as physiology and laboratory medicine had held back the development of the clinical school and allowed other centres to take advantage of a new focus on surgery and its attendant disciplines. While Acland claimed that his interests lay in promoting science in general and rejecting premature specialization, his outlook did appear to have serious consequences for Oxford science relative to Cambridge. Cambridge's 'moribund' medical school of the 1860s was turned around by the arrival of key personnel, Michael Foster and George Murray Humphrey (professor of anatomy from 1866). Yet even Humphrey acknowledged that Cambridge could not become a complete clinical school, and students continued their education in London. Acland was a key individual in the story of medical education at Oxford, and the 'lost medical school' debate has done much to damage his reputation, allowing him to become a scapegoat for those who were disappointed over the decline of the anatomy school.

In fact the nature of Oxford University made it difficult for the institution to respond to the changing emphasis within the medical curriculum. The experimental sciences had a growing dependence on extensive laboratory facilities, which, given the cost involved, could only be realized from a university-wide initiative. Wealth, in the Oxford system, resided within the colleges; the university lacked resources. Small residential colleges that emphasized individual learning based on a tutorial system were unlikely to need or desire such amenities. In 1873 George Rolleston, Linacre Professor of Anatomy and Physiology at Oxford, requested university finance to increase the remuneration and staffing of anatomy demonstrators in line with the amount allocated at Cambridge University. The latter spent £400 in this area against Oxford's £245.[24] Rolleston complained that there was little funding for microscopes. Acland and Rolleston were roundly criticized, but their position was a recognition that the will to create a true clinical school at the university was absent; as Acland complained, 'a practical school of medicine might be founded in Oxford; but the difficulties would be great and the cost enormous'.[25]

A debate about the future of medicine in Oxford began in the late 1870s within the ruling council of the university, and a series of meetings took place in 1879 which accepted evidence from influential medical men around the country. Lankester's position was unequivocal: 'there would be no practical difficulty in obtaining subjects for dissection for the teaching of human anatomy at Oxford, especially as at Cambridge they can be found for the purposes of as many as seventy students'.[26] He was largely, however, a lone voice. Acland and Rolleston were, by contrast, not alone in their opinion about medical education outside the metropolis. King Chambers, founder of St Mary's Medical School and the Royal Free Hospital, stated in his evidence given to a university committee examining the future of Oxford medicine:

> In the metropolis the student is, as it were, in a medical atmosphere, and he uncon-
> sciously imbibes a variety of notions which he digests and corrects by current
> observation of facts. The pupils of a provincial school are placed at a disadvantage
> by the isolation.[27]

Sir James Paget (1814–99)[28] did not think it would be wise to establish a medical school in Oxford. He felt that human anatomy could be introduced into
the arts course, but comparative anatomy was actually sufficient. He believed
that university education was only for those who would be teachers and readers and who could delay professional practice until the age of twenty-eight or
twenty-nine years. He wrote that Oxford should provide a preliminary general
education, 'educating young men to be gentlemen and men of science, who may
elsewhere be educated to be physicians and surgeons of the highest social and
practical rank'.[29] Sir William Gull (1816–90), Guy's Hospital physician, supported Acland's position on a broad science-based curriculum: he 'considers that
the attendance at hospital by undergraduates at Cambridge to be injurious'. A
key aspect of medical education was examined, and Professor Humphrey from
Cambridge said that 'sufficient subjects are obtained from a considerable area'
for his own medical school; but this was a problem for Oxford, as noted by Dr
Ogle: 'there is difficulty and great expense in procuring subjects'.[30]

As a result of these meetings and consultations, a final report was written by
Samuel West,[31] and he made his position clear from the opening line: 'Oxford
cannot have a complete medical school worthy of the University, and for this
reason, that it has not sufficient material for clinical instruction'. Although
the local hospital had the same number of beds as some London hospitals, he
supported Acland and recommended a solid scientific education in chemistry,
physics, botany and comparative anatomy, but 'complete clinical teaching of a
high order – of medicine, surgery, midwifery, gynaecology, ophthalmology –
[is] impossible in Oxford'.[32]

Professor Rolleston died in 1881, and the Linacre Professorship in Anatomy
and Physiology was divided up into the Linacre Chair in Human and Comparative Anatomy and the Waynflete Professorship in Physiology. In the same year
the Radcliffe Infirmary once again accepted six university students on the wards,
and new academic appointments gave a new impetus to the clinical aspects of
medical training at Oxford. By 1890 there were forty-three students walking
the wards. John Burdon-Sanderson, lately of University College London, as
Waynflete chair of physiology, and Arthur Thomson, from Edinburgh, as chair
of human anatomy, restored practical human anatomy as a separate academic
discipline at Oxford 'in the face of Acland's barely concealed disapproval'.[33] A
dedicated Faculty of Medicine opened in 1886, when Vice-Chancellor Jowett
(1817–93)[34] wrote to Florence Nightingale, 'the London medical world and
the Oxford, minus Dr Acland, approve the Statute'.[35] There were new academic

appointments, but expansion after 1880 was made very difficult by a continuing insistence on educating generalists of gentlemanly status rather than professional specialists. At the end of his career Acland reiterated his opinion that Oxford could not house a medical school:

> The term ... medical school is misleading ... if the school is to be of real repute it must be situated where material of all kinds and teachers in every branch can be had, abundantly and of the best, viz, in the great cities.[36]

John Burdon-Sanderson arrived in 1882 at Oxford as professor of physiology, and the struggles over funding for his elevated department illuminate the problems for 'scientific medicine' at the university. Burdon-Sanderson came to Oxford – with the support of Liddell (1811–98)[37] and Jowett, who were increasingly impatient of Acland – to establish a medical school and increase student numbers through the elevation of physiology. He was ultimately unsuccessful, due partly to the emphasis on gentlemanly pursuits over scientific excellence. Burdon-Sanderson moved to reform the examination system for medics at Oxford University as early as 1884, attempting to reduce the time required for a medical degree by decreasing the number of classical exams for undergraduates. He contacted Donald Macalister at Cambridge, who reported that the Cambridge medical degree counted towards the period of enrolment at the royal colleges and confirmed that some of the medical exams provided exemptions from college examination. Additionally, and key for Burdon-Sanderson, was the possibility of an award of a Cambridge medical degree within five years, while Oxford MDs still required eight years.

In 1885 Acland had received a letter from a father noting that he could not send his son to Oxford, 'not being able to afford to let him spend two preliminary years in pursuits which would be of little or no service to him'.[38] Burdon-Sanderson attempted to follow the Cambridge programme by shortening the Oxford degree and achieving recognition by the royal colleges. His demand for the abolition of moderations (the second of the classical examinations required at Oxford within the arts degree) was bound to cause difficulty: 'Acland has declared himself an opponent ... and would win'.[39] Burdon-Sanderson also proposed the exemption of students from parts of the Oxford degree course if they had passed the college conjoint examinations. This provision caused the greatest hostility within a newly organized group of Oxford graduates who made their opinions felt within the university hierarchy, and it was a key factor in Burdon-Sanderson's ultimate failure.

In 1884 a new Oxford medical graduates club was formed as a social group, but it became active within the hierarchy of the university almost at once. These graduates saw themselves as a small elite of medical practitioners, usually metropolitan consultants and teachers, who valued the time and money spent over their studies, and they viewed the conjoint scheme administered by the royal colleges as 'the *lowest standard* with which it is considered safe to let General Practitioners loose'.[40] They had no wish to increase the number of Oxford medical graduates, which, they believed, would devalue their own degrees. The graduates were very influential and allied with forces on Hebdomadal Council, some of whom were opposed to Burdon-Sanderson on anti-vivisection grounds, to have their views considered. The graduates were quick to remind Burdon-Sanderson that he was dependent on their support in council for his Physiology Department. As noted previously, the statute agreeing a new medical faculty was passed in 1885 but the examination system agreed by the colleges was not.

By the early 1890s Burdon-Sanderson noted a changing mood within the hierarchy of the university as finance for an anatomy building had been approved: 'the willingness with which this grant was voted affords the best evidence that it is no longer necessary to advocate the claim of medical science to be regarded as a university study'.[41] Acland was a spent force and was advised by Dean Liddell not to attend debates on funding for a new anatomy department in 1891.

> I have had letters from persons warmly attached to you and (I am sure) sincerely desirous of doing what is best for the study of medicine at Oxford. They deprecate in a most earnest and serious tone your intention of appearing in Convocation tomorrow as an active opponent of the Anatomical Scheme. They think that such an appearance would embitter your relations with those for whom you have worked so long and might end in your resignation – a remit which would be deeply regretted by all who know the enormous services which you have rendered to the cause of medical education in Oxford.[42]

Benjamin Jowett was one influential voice who was very critical of Acland, calling him 'one of the vainest, rudest men that ever lived' and stating, 'I believe him to be neither a man of science nor a good practitioner'.[43]

Burdon-Sanderson felt that the limited clinical experience available at the Radcliffe Infirmary could be overcome by sending students to the metropolitan hospitals. This was certainly the practice at Cambridge University. His major problem was the lack of staff available for teaching medics, as Acland had done nothing to increase teaching posts. There was no chair in pathology or pharmacology until the twentieth century, and Oxford was late in appointing staff to the discipline of physiology. Cambridge University, Owens College Manchester, King's and University College London, and Queens College Birmingham had all appointed physiology professors before Oxford. Burdon-Sanderson wanted to develop a dedicated Oxford University medical degree but was in conflict (somewhat ironically) with Lankester, who became Linacre Professor of Comparative Anatomy.[44] The latter demanded that undergraduates should be banned from attending human anatomy lectures. Arthur Thomson was a popular lecturer in anatomy, and Lankester believed that his demonstrations distracted students 'from more intellectually taxing work in pure biology'.[45] Liddell wrote in some surprise in March 1892: 'do I understand you to say Lankester wishes all Oxford medical graduates to go through the Arts course? If so, is he not merely taking a line in opposition to Sanderson'.[46]

In 1908 the vice-chancellor, T. H. Warren, regretted the decisions of the past: 'I have always held, and I think experience has justified the belief, that a strong medical school would be for the advantage of pure science at Oxford'.[47] The naissance of the new medical school at Oxford was paralleled by educational developments in Manchester, where the decline of the private medical school was arrested firstly by the establishment of Owens College and then by the Victoria University of Manchester.

Medical Education and Anatomy in Manchester

In the previous chapter the decline of the private medical school in Manchester was examined. Yet the school in Manchester survived, unlike several of the institutions that had been listed and licensed by the Anatomy Inspector in 1832. By 1858 institutions in Bath, Exeter, York and Hull had closed their doors to students, leaving schools in Bristol, Birmingham, Leeds, Liverpool, Manchester, Newcastle, Nottingham and Sheffield. The 1858 Medical Reform Act exacerbated the decline of the independent provincial anatomy school as it allowed the new General Medical Council to start restructuring the format of professional education. The council became increasingly concerned in the following decade over the basic standard of education for doctors, suggesting four years of study in one course over the traditional five-year apprenticeship. It also recommended that preclinical education should be dominated by practical anatomy and the study of the sciences favouring practical scientific training, including physiology and histology, demanding extensive laboratory facilities. This was an immediate problem for several schools (including Nottingham, which later closed as a result of these proposals).

Many provincial schools experienced a shortage of cadavers, which was extremely damaging at a time when anatomy was king, but they were able to develop a strong reputation in scientific pursuits, which was beneficial when other disciplines of laboratory medicine finally established a strong position within the medical curriculum. They could also claim large teaching hospitals: 'Metropolitan hospitals and medical schools stand pre-eminent, although of course, in some of our large towns, as Liverpool, Manchester, Birmingham or Bristol, there must be as much material for study'.[48]

Manchester's Owens College, founded in 1851, recognized the importance of preparing young men of the middle class for professional careers, and it had a strong focus on the classics and mathematics. The academic model was Oxford and Cambridge universities, although Owens was secular and catered for the sons of the Manchester middle class. Its founders refused to countenance a merger with the medical school, as the young medics were considered to be a poor influence on the more sensitive liberal arts students. The reputation of medicine in the 1850s can be illustrated by the refusal of Owens College to merge with the Manchester Medical School, despite the latter's royal title. Professor Williamson (1816–95) claimed that medical students would be

> a menace to the moral welfare of the normal arts and science students because medical students, and especially those in the provinces, were intellectually less sensitive and morally coarser than the average student and so would be a source of potential immorality.[49]

This was despite the fact that Williamson had been a student at Pine Street Anatomy School (1838–9), was a licentiate of the Society of Apothecaries and a member of the Royal College of Surgeons. His official title at Owens was professor of natural history, anatomy and physiology.[50] The medical men at the Royal School had wanted increased space to include a lecture room, museum, dissecting room and students' room as well as an attendant. Owens staff saw little in it for the college (even some of those in favour of union wanted segregation of the medical students).

Within a few years, however, Owens College was in severe financial difficulty and saw the solution in providing strong scientific education by recruiting key personnel. H. E. Roscoe (1833–1915), the professor of chemistry appointed in 1859, built 'the biggest and very probably the best school of chemistry in the country'.[51] In 1861 Robert Clifton was appointed to teach physics. The Owens hierarchy realized that a merger with the medical school would provide a ready market for its science courses. There was another chance at union in 1866, and by then the college could see that a medical faculty would help claims for university status. The two institutions merged in 1872, and Roscoe and the head of the medical school, George Southam, toured the London medical schools in order to plan the new medical school. In the following year money was found for a chair in physiology occupied by Arthur Gamgee (1841–1909), and the new medical school buildings were opened shortly after. The new chair was appointed to research and teach and was precluded from clinical practice. This rule was extended to all anatomy and pathology teachers appointed in the next five years.

The education of surgeons and physicians was increasingly based on a common course of study still heavily dominated by anatomy but encompassing new laboratory sciences that needed to be located within university-type institutions. The failure of the traditional universities to provide adequate medical education was one spur for the development of alternatives outside of the supply in Scotland, notably Manchester. George Paget (1809–92),[52] Regius Professor of Physic at Cambridge, noted that 'there were loud complaints outside that

Oxford and Cambridge do little or nothing for medicine, and this fact provided the chief argument for the establishment of one or two northern universities.'[53] This was supported by an 1882 Royal Commission which recommended that Owens College be given its own degree-awarding powers.[54]

A university charter was granted to Owens College in 1880, and medical degrees continued to be awarded by the University of London (Manchester students had been able to take the London University exams since 1859). The Victoria University consisted of Owens, University College of Liverpool (1884) and the Yorkshire College of Leeds (1887). Medical degrees awarded by the Victoria University were not available until 1904: 'A memorial drawn up and signed by a considerable number of the members of the medical profession, prayed that the right of conferring medical degrees might not be granted to the Victoria University', as there were already nineteen authorized corporations and there was a belief that competition 'tends to lower the standard of medical qualification.'[55]

Almost immediately, however, it was apparent that the pursuit of medicine was neglected by the existing English universities. John Morgan, professor of medicine at the Victoria University and honorary physician at the Manchester Royal Infirmary, asserted that 63 per cent of Scottish medical men had degrees and Ireland could boast 30 per cent, while in England only 5 per cent of doctors held degrees.[56] Morgan noted that the Victoria University had a key claim to degree-awarding status as an alternative to Oxford and Cambridge:

> Although many subjects bearing upon medicine may be admirably taught in the old universities, as has been so well exemplified at Cambridge during the last eight or ten years; still a complete course of medical training seems incompatible with the restricted opportunities for clinical observation which such comparatively small towns as Oxford and Cambridge can supply to the student.[57]

Additionally, Morgan maintained that the Victoria University was 'a University specially founded for the hard-working middle classes, from among whose ranks the representatives of medicine are almost solely recruited.'[58]

Owens College in Manchester was singled out in *The Medical Student's Guide* of 1876: 'the new building contains every convenience for medical education.'[59] The prospectus for the Victoria University of Manchester Medical School for 1908 makes much of the dissection material available for second-year students:

> If there is one point which stands out most prominently in the many conspicuous recommendations of the Manchester Medical School, it is the wealth of material – anatomical, pathological, and clinical – at the disposal of the teachers, and this has been a characteristic feature during the whole of its career. One of the greatest difficulties of medical schools is to obtain a sufficient supply of subjects for dissection, but this has never been felt at Manchester ... There is accommodation in the dissecting room for 250 students.[60]

One 1885 guide for medical students noted that 'Manchester possesses one of the largest and most important of the provincial schools of medicine and that the degree of the Victoria University is likely to rank high'.[61] Just seven years earlier the guide had reported that 'two persons out of three who have been educated wholly at a provincial school are ashamed of it'.[62]

Henry Acland certainly recognized the growing importance of the northern colleges and saw that Oxford could not compete in clinical training. He was concerned that Oxford 'will run a risk of losing its character as a scientific institution ... if it attempts to rival the great metropolitan schools or the Victoria University, it will fail'.[63] Owens was certainly ambitious, and it was the second institution in England to appoint a full-time professor of physiology (second only to Cambridge, with Michael Foster). The appointment of Arthur Gamgee was made in 1873, ten years before Oxford's appointment of John Burdon-Sanderson as Waynflete Professor of Physiology. Part of Manchester's eventual success in medical education was due to an ability to secure bodies through parochial authorities and also through the city's voluntary hospitals, which not only provided post-mortem examinations but allowed students to link anatomy to clinical care. The rest of this chapter studies the relationship between medical education and the hospital, focusing more closely on the experience in Oxford.

Hospital Medical Education in Oxford

Surgery was not part of the academic medical course at Oxford University, although surgeons assisted in anatomical dissections and had their own apprentices who could attend the infirmary. Between 1780 and 1800 the number of Oxford medical students doubled, and half later became fellows of the Royal College of Physicians. In 1839 the infirmary held over 140 beds and Alexander Robb-Smith claims that 'accordingly the Infirmary was one of the institutions where a student might put in a part of the surgical and the whole of the medical portion of his training'.[64] There were three types of pupil: students introduced by individual surgeons and physicians; Oxford medical students; and non-professional students at the university aiming to qualify as clergymen or missionaries. The students attended lectures and instruction in anatomy, physiology, chemistry, materia medica, medicine, midwifery, surgery, botany and forensic medicine. In 1840 the Weekly Board of the Infirmary reiterated its role as a clinical school of medical education. The Board duly divided the educational year into winter and summer sessions in response to the Apothecaries Company regulations of 1835:

> The Weekly Board [is] anxious to forward the wishes of the Governors in general and to make their Infirmary available under proper regulations for the Professional Education not only of the Students in medicine belonging to the University, but also of young men intended to be surgeons, apothecaries, and general practitioners.[65]

The Radcliffe Infirmary went into severe decline as a clinical medical school during the nineteenth century partly as a result of the overhaul of the examination system by the university, much of which was carried out by Acland. The 1850 Royal Commission on the Universities recognized the role of Oxford in conferring future social status at the expense of clinical teaching:

> Oxford has ceased altogether to be a school of medicine. Those few persons who take medical degrees there with a view to the social consideration which these degrees give, or the preferments in the University for which they are necessary, study their profession elsewhere.[66]

Between 1837 and 1840 there were thirty-seven pupils of the university attached to the Radcliffe Infirmary under Regius Professor Ogle. When Acland became clinical professor, he taught the last twelve students at the Radcliffe. The clinical professor during the 1830s and 1840s, Ogle believed that the lack of interest in clinical medicine was inevitable given the size of Oxford; yet Cambridge managed to retain a small clinical school at Addenbrooke's Hospital, where there was a greater willingness to adapt teaching to the needs of preclinical medical students who needed to meet the licensing requirements of the GMC. By the 1880s there were around eighty clinical students at Addenbrooke's Hospital, a policy that had been fostered by men such as Michael Foster. The 1876 *Medical Student's Guide* noted that the Radcliffe Infirmary held over 160 beds but no medical school.[67]

One medical student wrote to the *British Medical Journal* reporting his request to Acland to undertake clinical study at the Radcliffe Infirmary:

> The Clinical Professor raised no objection to my studying at the Radcliffe Infirmary, but said that he had never given certificates for such study, and that he would give none to me ... Imagine the consternation that would be caused at Cambridge or Trinity College, Dublin, by a similar discouragement on the part of the Regius Professor of Physic from clinical study within the walls of his own hospital.

Glynn Whittle worked in the surgical wards of the Radcliffe Infirmary without gaining a certificate but felt that there were 'just as good opportunities for clinical work as any other hospital of the same size'.[68]

The numbers of non-university students, those undertaking medical studies by apprenticeship, also severely declined just a few years after the infirmary conformed to the rules of the Apothecaries Society. In March 1846 a letter from Mr Westell, a gentleman of Witney and guardian to Mr Sheppard, the infirmary's own apprentice surgeon-apothecary, caused some concern to the Board, as Mr Westell requested the early termination of Mr Sheppard's appointment. If the young man was to satisfy the requirements of the College of Surgeons and Apothecaries Hall, 'it is indispensable that he shall have attended certain lectures *in London* during *three sessions* at one or more of the metropolitan hospitals'. Mr Westell said it was imperative for his ward to start in London in October, 'or he will be ineligible for examination until after an age when he cannot by the regulations of the Service, enter the Navy for which he is intended'.[69] Increasingly as the century wore on, the two official medical bodies, the Society of Apothecaries and the Royal College of Surgeons, emphasized the importance of clinical training in London and allowed for shorter periods of attendance on the wards at the London hospitals, in preference to provincial hospitals.

Cambridge University made some efforts to develop clinical medical education. In 1842 George Paget introduced the first practical examination for medical students at Addenbrooke's Hospital, where patients had to be examined and treatments discussed in front of an examiner. Paget and George Humphrey began clinical lectures at the hospital in the following year. There was, however, an eventual recognition that the clinical school would always be limited, relying on a strong link with the London medical schools. As professor of physic, Paget was ultimately disappointed in his aims to introduce new areas of clinical medicine into the Cambridge curriculum, notably medical jurisprudence, midwifery and public health. Professor Humphrey was concerned that money should not be frittered away on 'the establishment of poorly paid professorships' in efforts to become 'a second rate medical school'.[70] The focus remained on the first few years of medical education. The *British Medical Journal* reported in 1883 that Cambridge 'is and must remain a School to be frequented chiefly in the first two or three years of a student's career ... great clinical schools can only exist in great centres of population'.[71]

While clinical opportunities were not exploited, it is tempting to speculate that provincial areas such as Oxford and Cambridge may have relied more on the hospital post-mortem to provide teaching opportunities when bodies were scarce through the usual channels. Unusually some post-mortem records from the Radcliffe Infirmary have survived, although they must be treated with care as they are heavily annotated and in poor condition. Table IV in the Appendix gives the numbers of deaths at the Radcliffe Infirmary over the century and the number of attendant post-mortems. It is interesting to note that there was a large number of post-mortems conducted just around the time of a new impetus within Oxford anatomy with the arrival of new personnel (see Chapter 4), and that there were very few in the period immediately preceding this. Of course, many of these post-mortems were no doubt conducted at the behest of the coroner and not through any great interest from clinicians, although there was certainly much post-mortem anatomizing in the 1840s as well. The numbers were extremely low in the middle of the century, with little interest from either clinicians or the coroner. There is evidence that relatives refused permission and these are duly noticed, but what is striking is how few these are.

Despite the criticism directed at Acland, at the end of his career he was certainly not alone in his opinion that towns such as Oxford and Cambridge were at a distinct disadvantage in providing necessary clinical material for medical students. However, his position regarding liberal education for generalists was out of step with increasing demands for cheaper and more accessible scientific medical education. Acland lamented the dominance of sciences alone within the medical curriculum: 'The course of things has lately tended to drive Oxford men prepared for the great profession of medicine out of the ranks of literary, historical or philosophical culture'.[72]

Hospital Medical Education in Manchester

The great claim for any medical course in addition to large numbers of cadavers, as evidenced by John Morgan's attitude, was the access to clinical medical cases in the local hospital. Morgan noted that the Victoria University was in a 'densely-populated' region (as opposed to the Radcliffe Infirmary and Addenbrooke's, which were in areas of 'sparse rural population').[73] In Manchester, however, there was an initial problem as all the local voluntary hospitals were extremely concerned over a possible clash between clinical teaching and the desire to care for the sick poor. The Manchester Royal Infirmary in particular fought against medical school control. Additionally, Owens College refused to guarantee to appoint professors from the staff of the infirmary. At University College and King's College in London, hospitals had grown up around the medical schools. The other London schools grew out of hospitals. This did not occur in the same way outside of London. The clinical professor at Owens College in 1888 was temporarily unable to gain access to the infirmary and gave his lectures at the more limited Ancoats hospital. The control over clinical beds at the Manchester Royal Infirmary was a contentious issue that led ultimately to victory for the medical school.

Conclusion

This chapter has taken a broad look at medical education in the later nineteenth century (demanded by the Medical Reform Act). The increasing acceptance of medical education based on the specialized medical school, focused firstly on anatomy and later on physiology and pathology, and linked to the observation and experience available at large hospitals, cast a poor light on the education available at the English universities with their concentration on ancient texts. Michael Foster found that the rising men of the medical profession were no longer necessarily from the two English universities and that in future Oxbridge graduates would be 'an insignificant minority'.[74] The proximity of London University to the major metropolitan hospitals gave it a huge advantage in attracting medical students, although Oxbridge held onto a major benefit until 1854, when the London medical degree could finally be used as a licence to practise medicine. Until then London medical students still had to qualify through the Royal College of Surgeons or the Society of Apothecaries, unlike alumni of Oxford and Cambridge.

Oxford University could have adapted along the lines followed by Cambridge, but the people in key positions, namely Acland and Rolleston, held no great belief in undergraduate clinical medicine, preferring to concentrate on science and allowing medics to continue their studies in London. In 1884 the English Conjoint Board was set up as the examining board for both of the royal colleges, physicians and surgeons, providing the MRCS, LRCP and a licence for general practice. In the following year doctors, by order of the General Medical Council, had to undergo a five-year common medical course, a regulation that was adopted by most institutions, including Cambridge University. Oxford University continued to insist that a medical degree took eight years to achieve, but compromised down to seven years in 1887.

The key medical personnel at Oxford University persisted in regarding the increasing emphasis on specialization with suspicion, but it also suffered as an institution that found change difficult. Power and wealth at the university resided in the colleges, resulting in inertia over the funding of expensive university-wide laboratories and staff. However, the key to the best medical education was the linking of academic theory to the clinical opportunities only available within a large hospital. In this setting, medical students could attend lectures and demonstrations and then visit the patients on the ward, finally tracing the unsuccessful cases right through to the mortuary, furthering their education through post-mortem examination. As noted, this feature could well have overcome the difficulty of finding bodies in the anatomy lectures.[75]

Oxford University suffered in medical education at a time when university education was largely irrelevant for the bulk of medical practitioners. Surgery was on the rise, with anatomy as its key skill. This subject was best taught in small groups in the private anatomical schools that sprung up in London and other large towns. Access to bodies was vital. Yet the dominance of the private schools, so well suited to minute dissection, was short-lived, giving way once more to the large university and attendant teaching hospital. Richardson was correct in noting that private schools lost out to hospitals, but the Royal College of Surgeons was a driving force in protecting the vested interests of its teachers at those hospital schools and moved against the private schools. Manchester was certainly affected by this, and the protracted argument is outlined in Chapter 1. Even with the interference of the royal college, the infirmary at Manchester had a far greater claim to metropolitan status than the Radcliffe Infirmary in Oxford, which made no attempt to become a recognized clinical school until the twentieth century.

Manchester's private medical school went into a severe decline in the middle of the nineteenth century, but it recovered sufficiently at the end of the century to join forces with the increasingly respected Owens College. This was a key strategy for the survival of other independent provincial medical schools.[76] The Manchester unification was considered with suspicion at first by Owens professors, who considered medical students as socially inferior to the college's traditional alumni. The local medical student was almost wholly concerned with anatomy and surgery and was tainted for some time with this association. However, the changing nature of medical training demanded by the General Medical Council brought Owens around to the idea that a strong association with the medical school would add weight to their own demands for university status and supply much-needed students for science courses. The eventual union provided the impetus for the college to form the Victoria University. The General Medical Council had by this time come to demand the end of apprenticeships and private courses and to elevate the university course, not just for physicians but for all medical disciplines. The new civic universities were popular institutions for the provincial middle class, which could send their sons into well-respected professions without the huge cost of metropolitan training and the temptations of the capital. The popularity of the Owens College medical school led to a decrease in London medical schools in the last two decades of the nineteenth century and London University's attempts to restructure the medical degree.

6 SOME CONTEMPORARY PARALLELS

The deep-seated fear over the post-mortem use of human body parts remains a concern in the modern era, despite the increasing secularization of society and new developments in medical science. The perceived acceptance of invasive forms of medicine – particularly procedures within surgery, notably transplantation – does not secure medics from approbation when they are seen to operate outside the bounds of socially accepted boundaries. However, the issue is not clear-cut; as well as public outrage after revelations by the media, there is also widespread interest in the anatomy of the human body.

Anatomy Teaching

Anatomy teaching and the use of bodies by medical schools has become an area that is less controversial; most medical schools no longer require preclinical medical students to dissect cadavers but instead use prosection specimens for teaching anatomy, while current preservation techniques enable bodies and body parts to be retained for many years. The very small numbers of current donations are sufficient for use. While anatomical dissection is no longer a part of undergraduate medical education, it is still an essential element of postgraduate training for surgeons. As access to cadavers has been reduced, acquiring expertise in anatomy and dissection is facilitated by the use of anatomy models, radiographic techniques and computer-assisted learning.

Pathology emerged as an important area of medical teaching in the late nineteenth century. Teaching pathology to clinical medical students requires preserved organs demonstrating various diseases and utilizes pathology pots. Pathology pots are held in pathology museums in many medical schools, and large collections were built up until the 1970s. Since then there have been few new specimens made – most teaching today uses specimens that are up to one hundred years old. Some of the large collections are now of historical importance in addition to being valuable teaching resources for medical students, such as the museum at Guy's Hospital. A small number are open to the public, for instance the Hunterian Collection at the Royal College of Surgeons in London.

Since the institution of the Retained Organ Commission in 2001, many specimens have been destroyed. Others have been locked away, reducing access to medical students. In an attempt to preserve existing specimens for the teaching of future medical students, the Royal College of Pathologists is developing an online resource of pathology pots.

There remains a need to teach trainee pathologists, again as a postgraduate activity that necessitates access to fresh cadavers for post-mortem examination. Whereas previously these were provided by consented hospital post-mortems, with the demise of the consented autopsy, autopsies requested by coroners are now the major teaching resource for pathologists and medical students. The reasons for a reduction in consented autopsies are various, but key must be the organ retention scandals of the 1990s, notably Bristol and Alder Hey (discussed further below), which consequently led to the creation of the Retained Organ Commission and the Human Tissue Authority. The HTA was created in 2004 and began operating two years later; its remit is to regulate the removal, storage, use and disposal of human bodies, organs and tissues for research, transplantation and education. The establishment of the HTA meant the abolition of the post of HM Inspector of Anatomy. The retention of tissue by medical schools requires consent from the HTA, and this is lacking for many specimens that pre-date 2004.

Bodies are available for examination through the coroner's service. Just as in the eighteenth and nineteenth centuries, it is the function of the coroner to investigate unexpected deaths, and so there is often a requirement for autopsy. The autopsy aims to identify cause of death and collect information for inquest. Coronial law has resulted in a high autopsy rate (22 per cent of deaths) in England and Wales, higher than in most other countries. There have been strong religious objections to the coroner's autopsy that have grown in influence in recent years. Muslim and Jewish communities have requested a non-invasive alternative, and this led to a private post-mortem radiology service being set up in Manchester in 1990s, based on scanning bodies. The Department of Health and the Royal College of Pathologists have set up a joint working group that is currently drafting recommendations for teaching and detailing validation and accreditation documents for post-mortem imaging acceptable for death certification purposes.

The use of body parts in education is now heavily regulated for medical professionals. There is also, however, a thirst for knowledge of anatomy and medicine within the general public, and the presentation of this occupies a very grey area between education and entertainment.

Body Worlds

In 2002 the Body Worlds exhibition opened in London to fascination and revulsion in equal measure. It was set up by anatomist Gunther von Hagens, who had invented a process known as plastination, developed in Heidelberg between 1977 and 1982. As a result of the success of the exhibition, von Hagens conducted the first public autopsy in the United Kingdom for 170 years. It was attended by 500 people, happy to be an audience in the manner of the public dissections of the seventeenth century. Von Hagens conducted the demonstration wearing his trademark fedora hat, echoing the dress style of the old anatomists pictured in the paintings of the old masters. He had received a letter from Her Majesty's Inspector of Anatomy warning that the autopsy would be a criminal act under section eleven of the 1984 Anatomy Act. One hundred and thirty complaints were received by Channel 4, which screened the act, but no action was ultimately taken. Since 1995, when von Hagens first staged his exhibition in Tokyo, Body Worlds has become big business. Von Hagens employs 340 people at five laboratories in four countries plastinating bodies for display in exhibitions, and his television appearances continue. It is possible to purchase a document at Body Worlds exhibitions detailing the procedure for donating one's body for plastination. Von Hagens's latest business venture has been to offer body parts for sale online, including plastinated 'slices' of corpses, much to the anger of Christians in his native Germany.[1]

The parallels in the work of von Hagens with the behaviour of past anatomists are striking. In February 2004 the *Suddeutsche Zietung* reported that von Hagens had offered a payment and pension to Alexander Sizonenko if the latter would agree to have his body plastinated after death. Sizonenko was 2.39 metres (7 feet 10 inches) tall. Sizonenko declined the offer and died in 2012.[2] Pursuing a particular body was something that anatomists had done since the eighteenth century: in 1792 the 'tallest man in the world', Charles Byrne, arrived in London and put himself on public display. Within a year it was obvious that the twenty-one-year-old was dying. His greatest fear was that his body would end up on an anatomist's table. He arranged for his friends to seal his body in a lead coffin, watch over it for four days, and then drop the coffin into the sea. Hunter had, however, bribed the undertaker, and the corpse of the giant ended up in Hunter's possession. The skeleton formed a key exhibit in the Hunterian Museum. Hunter claimed he had paid the huge sum of one hundred and thirty guineas for the body, but it was rumoured to be a great deal more.[3] Presumably von Hagens was less successful in his quest.

Von Hagens has not always escaped public approbation and official reaction. He was once forced to return controversial corpses to China in 2004. Von Hagens has never been clear about where the corpses for his plastination work originated, although he claims that many are bequeathed, and on this occasion seven may actually have come from executed prisoners. As reported in the *Guardian*, the German magazine *Der Spiegel* had discovered that at least two of the 647 corpses stored at one of von Hagens's centres in China had bullet holes in their skulls. It was claimed that an email from Sui Hongjin, his manager in China, said that Sui had obtained bodies of a young man and young woman in December 2001; they had died that morning, and thus they were 'fresh examples' of 'highest quality'. The *Guardian* continued: 'The centre is close to three prison camps, which are home to political detainees and members of the banned Falun Gong movement. According to Amnesty International, China's communist authorities executed 2,468 people in 2001 by shooting them in the head or the back of the neck. Prof von Hagens has previously been accused of buying the corpses of prisoners, homeless people and the mentally ill in Russia – a charge he denies'.[4]

Von Hagens has often found himself in the same sort of controversy and intrigue that arose before and immediately after the passing of the 1832 Anatomy Act in England. In 2002 a pathologist and coroner in Siberia was charged with criminal proceedings over a shipment of fifty-six corpses on their way to Heidelberg.[5] Police said the Novosibirsk coroner, Vladimir Novosylow, had sold the bodies, but ultimately von Hagens was not actually charged in the case. The police instituted an investigation in Kyrgyzstan into the plastination of hundreds of corpses from prisons and psychiatric hospitals without notification to their families. Again the accusations were strongly denied by von Hagens in the 'Statement on Wrongful Allegations and False Reports by Media on the Origin of Bodies in BODY WORLDS Exhibition', a press release from his Institut fur Plastination, 4 March 2006.

Eighteenth- and nineteenth-century anatomists were often accused of turning a blind eye to the sources of corpses, even when it later seemed obvious that the victims may have been murdered. Dr Knox, the Edinburgh anatomist at the centre of the Burke and Hare murders, was forced to leave his practice in the city and to set up in London after the reaction of the local population.

In a 2011 article titled 'Physician Plastinate Thyself', the *Independent* newspaper revealed that von Hagens was suffering from Parkinson's disease and planned to leave instructions for his own plastination.[6] Few anatomists in the past have allowed their own bodies to be used for dissection purposes after death. John Hunter was a notable exception, but his brother William, equally famed as an anatomist, made sure his own body was buried in a secure vault.

Organ Retention Scandals – Bristol and Liverpool

The work of von Hagens illustrates the contradiction between the public fascination of anatomy and the underlying fear of the anatomists' source material. The 1990s pathology scandal, which first broke at the Bristol Royal Infirmary and then widened to Alder Hey Hospital and other centres, demonstrated a more immediate and general fear of the work of surgeons and pathologists, with no accompanying interest in the work of anatomy.

Between 1988 and 1995 two surgeons at the Bristol Royal Infirmary performed very challenging arterial switch operations on babies' hearts. Thirty-five children died as a result of these and other heart operations. The arterial procedure was new and was performed on critically ill children, but the death rate was considered to be high, and the surgeons became the subject of the allegations of medical malpractice. The tragedy was compounded for the affected parents by the discovery that children's hearts had been retained by the pathologists undertaking the autopsies, which were required for all deaths occurring on the operating table:

> My blood just ran cold. Samantha's surgeon was at the centre of the allegations of malpractice. I immediately demanded a copy of her medical records from the hospital. I found myself staring at a letter from the pathologist who performed the post-mortem to her surgeon, stating that he had retained the heart. I was horrified and felt bitterly angry that this had happened without my knowledge. Organ retention without consent was routine practice and I didn't know who my daughter's heart belonged to – me or the hospital's pathology department.[7]

In February 1999 the hospital confirmed that it had retained the hearts from over 170 children from 1983 to 1995. It was later revealed that 11,000 hearts were being stored nationwide.[8] For those interested in the Bristol case, Tim Marshall's work *Stolen Hearts: Fiction and the 1990s' Pathology Scandal* gives a clear outline of the problems encountered when introducing innovative surgery without a culture of honesty within medical institutions.

What is of key concern here is the escalation of the scandal once it was realized that body parts were kept by clinicians without the permission (whether legally necessary or not) or even knowledge of relatives. The formal inquiry into the Bristol scandal was told in 1999 that Alder Hey Children's Hospital in Liverpool had a very large collection of hearts taken from 800 children, largely by Professor Dick van Velzen, consultant pathologist. The resulting investigation revealed that van Velzen was not alone in taking body parts without consent, and there were around 105,000 body parts stored in British hospitals. The legal issue over ownership of the body is unclear, as it was in the eighteenth and nineteenth centuries, but doctors certainly believed that there was no compulsion to ask for permission to take body parts as part of a post-mortem examination. Most post-mortems in the United Kingdom are conducted under orders from the coroner, and relatives cannot object to post-mortems under this legal framework. There are relatively few hospital post-mortems conducted. This may reflect a reluctance of clinicians to request them, in part due to fears of relatives' reactions as well as the increased administrative burden since the pathology scandals of the recent past. The decline of the hospital post-mortem may have unfortunate long-term consequences for medical education and quality of clinical care, as autopsy findings play an important role in clinical audit.

What transpired during the recent organ retention inquiries was a realization that relatives were unaware of the implications of post-mortem and that the taking of 'tissues' could often mean whole organs stored for very long periods of time. The report, published in 2001, contained much that had startling parallels with the activities of anatomists in the past, as revealed in the nineteenth-century records from the Anatomy Inspectorate. What is most obvious is that while the present-day activities that gave rise to the scandals were not illegal, many doctors were still acting in a very secretive manner, fearing that too much knowledge of their actions would result in a public outcry. In 1999 one family expressed their horror at discovering that their son's body was buried without his heart; his mother, Daphne Ford, said that she felt as 'if it was stolen'.[9]

As detailed above, many find the thought of their loved ones' bodies being opened and dissected extremely distressing, and some faith groups, notably the Jewish and Muslim communities, have religious objections. There is public demand for an alternative to invasive autopsy, and as a result the Department of Health has allocated funding to investigate whether imaging has the greatest potential to detect the wide range of conditions that can cause death. Ian Roberts, professor of cellular pathology in Oxford, and his colleagues have conducted post-mortems and scans on 182 bodies in Oxford and Manchester to date.[10] The work is not yet complete, but the initial findings are encouraging. In the future it may be possible to establish cause of death from imaging techniques, leaving the body undisturbed.

Nineteenth-century dissection took place on a body, regardless of cause or nature of death, to demonstrate anatomy to medical students. Large numbers were needed. Today, due to our ability to preserve the body from putrefaction, the small number of bequests meets the need of students and there are no shortages (although this might be set to change in the light of increasing suspicion of the medical profession caused by the organ retention scandals). Today the shortage of bodies resides within the area of the hospital post-mortem required for the teaching of morbid anatomy – the changes in the body in association with disease.[11] These consented autopsies are required for demonstration of diseased organs to medical students and for the training of specialists in hospital medicine, surgery and pathology. The great majority of autopsies today are performed for medicolegal reasons on the instruction of the coroner, in order to determine the cause of sudden unexpected deaths or to investigate potentially unnatural deaths, rather than for teaching purposes. The Anatomy Act of 1832 had a profound effect on medical education in the regions as it failed to realize the numbers of cadavers needed by students. Current legislation and attitudes may have equally important implications for the future development of medical education in the UK.

CONCLUSION

Oxford, Manchester and the Anatomy Act

The growing affluence of the middle and working classes led to a demand for cheaper, more accessible medical care. The providers of this were the new breed of general practitioners whose grounding was in surgery, and their training was largely provided by the London and provincial anatomy schools. Detailed anatomy was, for most nineteenth-century medical men, a skill rarely called upon in general practice. It was, however, a crucial element in doctors' claims to respectability and status, as it was central to their identity as men of science. Doctors found that anatomical proficiency was a means of distancing themselves from 'quacks' at a time when there was little uniform medical training or qualification. The elevation of anatomy necessitated a supply of bodies, which was only realized firstly from the gallows and latterly from a widespread trade in bodysnatching. Again, claims to be men of professional standards led doctors to demand a more respectable source of dissection material. Medical men were tainted by their strong link to the degraded and hated resurrection men.

The 1832 Anatomy Act was an effort by Parliament to provide an adequate supply of cadavers for independent anatomy schools, which had become the lynchpin of medical education in the late eighteenth century. Anatomy allowed medical men of all disciplines to claim expertise and status despite little advance in therapeutics. The nineteenth century saw the marginal position of medical men improve and their own insecurity give way to greater professional self-confidence and a belief in the advancement of medical science. This self-confidence was rooted in a claim to be men of science and could be used to demand status and autonomy. The *Edinburgh Medical and Surgical Journal* expressed concern over men who were 'engaged in the trading, money-making parts of the profession, and not one in a hundred of them distinguished by anything like science or liberality of mind'.[1] The development of dedicated anatomical language was an important aspect of the claims of doctors to professional and educated expertise. As a result their education became increasingly rooted in the specialized medical school, focused firstly on anatomy and later in physiology and pathology, linked to observation and experience available at large hospitals.

It has been necessary to examine medical education from an early period well before the passing of the Anatomy Act, outlining the rise of public anatomical investigation during the Renaissance and investigating the supply of bodies to anatomists. This research demonstrates that bodysnatching was prevalent beyond the metropolitan centres of London and Edinburgh, as regional centres had their own medical students and gangs interested in raising the dead for study. Oxford anatomists were recipients of bodies from the gallows around the city, although numbers were very small. There is some evidence that the anatomists at the university utilized the trade in bodysnatching. Manchester was a key location in the body trade, benefiting the city's anatomists and others around the country. This research demonstrates the extent of bodysnatching in the city and its involvement in supplying other centres, notably Edinburgh.

Effects of the Anatomy Act on Body Supply

Oxford University certainly never managed to secure a decent supply of cadavers through the Anatomy Act, and it largely abandoned the teaching of anatomy for much of the nineteenth century. The university educated elite physicians and failed to adapt to the new anatomically focused medical education, which elevated the role of the socially inferior surgeon. The Oxford system made change difficult, as power was located within the small and largely autonomous colleges. Expensive new medical facilities were difficult to institute on a university-wide basis. The contention in the present research accepts to a limited extent Richardson's point that Oxford also suffered from few available bodies for dissection. The city was small, and most people had family and friends prepared to bury them. The city was in any case dominated by a clerical elite disposed towards the respectable burial of the poor. Cambridge University also experienced this problem but managed to build up a more successful anatomy school due to the keen efforts of several dedicated individuals. The staff of the Oxford school showed no similar enthusiasm, and the study of anatomy became moribund at Oxford for much of the nineteenth century, as students relied on their proximity to London for the completion of anatomical and clinical studies within the large teaching hospitals.

The Manchester anatomy schools were more committed and successful in securing bodies, but they gave way to the consolidation of medical teaching within one pre-eminent institution that ultimately amalgamated university and hospital teaching. The demise of the independent schools is not simply the result of body shortage. Hospital-based schools were certainly in a much better position to provide medical training by providing educational material from the bedside through to the mortuary, thereby instituting a vital link between clinical medicine and post-mortem. In Manchester bodies were more readily available, but there were periodic shortages which were noted by the Anatomy Inspector, who also berated the existence of multiple schools within one locality. The Royal College of Surgeons had never approved of the teaching of anatomy outside of their own favoured metropolitan institutions. Small provincial schools struggled to get their teachers and courses recognized, and those that were unsuccessful inevitably failed, regardless of body numbers.

Wider Significance of the Anatomy Act – Attitudes to the Poor

There is some evidence of concern over dissection and care of the dead within Manchester and Oxford in the period just prior to the passing of the Anatomy Act. There are examples of disturbances at public executions in Oxford and a possibility that in Oxford and Manchester riots associated with agricultural and electoral change were bound up with an array of grievances, including dissection and anatomy. The work analyses the known anatomy riots as well as those associated with enclosure in Otmoor and cholera in Manchester to illustrate the multi-layered nature of public disturbance. The extensive examination of Hansard is a new attempt to illustrate that public disquiet over anatomy was often hidden from public view because of the furore over the passing of the Reform Act.

The passing of the Anatomy Act did not result in large numbers of bodies becoming available. This research indicates that there was no great change in attitudes within the selected localities to the burial of the poor, even when the individuals concerned were obviously unclaimed and unlamented.

There is overwhelming evidence to suggest that the Oxford University professors struggled to secure a reasonable supply of bodies when demands for cadavers were increasing. Local workhouses did not release bodies to the anatomists and preferred to bury the bodies at rate-payers' expense. Manchester, as a larger city, contained several successful anatomy schools, but there is evidence that the supply did not remain secure, and there is much correspondence in the anatomy records to indicate that parochial authorities often viewed anatomists with suspicion and buried the poor at public expense.

There is certainly little evidence from Manchester or Oxford to show a particular concern for the passing of the Anatomy Act, and the evidence actually suggests that there was no great enthusiasm from parochial authorities for giving up bodies of the poor to anatomists. However, it must be noted that there has always been a suspicion between the poor and the medical profession, and much of this is based on a concern over surgery and anatomy. The *Lancet* reported that 'We have reason to believe that it is not an uncommon practice for paupers in workhouses to bequeath their bodies to fellow inmates to prevent their being utilized for dissection under the Anatomy Act'.[2] This is a fascinating comment, but regrettably the views of workhouse residents were rarely recorded. There are strong indications continuing throughout the late nineteenth and early twentieth centuries (and indeed up to the present) that post-mortem examination, which usually took place in hospitals (including workhouse infirmaries), became the major focus for widespread suspicion. In 1896 the *Lancet* informed doctors that 'it is illegal to make a post-mortem examination without the permission of the friends of a deceased person, or the Coroner'.[3] Without permission, the post-mortem was 'an assault upon the body'.

There was often surprise articulated within the medical profession that 'the silly old prejudice against post-mortem examinations' had not died out. The *Lancet* expressed frustration that the example of 'the educated classes' had not managed to dispel the 'dense ignorance of the lower orders'.[4] In 1904, on taking up his new office, the Manchester coroner reported:

> practically no bodies were sent to mortuaries even for post-mortem work. When first I introduced the habit of removing them in the case of post-mortems there were riots in the streets sometimes, and when I sent my officers to remove a body, in one or two cases the friends of the deceased rallied and rescued the body and took it away. Very great tact has been required to get matters as far as I have got them.[5]

The *Lancet* reported in 1909 of a Manchester widow who said she had been intimidated by the doctor into giving permission for a post-mortem on her husband, who had died in the workhouse. The *Lancet* defended the doctor, stating that he had been concerned about typhoid and had mistakenly told the widow that a post-mortem must take place. He did this 'accidentally and in the interests of the institution'. One woman guardian had objected that too many post-mortems were taking place at Chorlton Workhouse: 'the Hospital should not be a practising ground for young doctors'. The *Lancet* editorial wrote:

> It is a pity to see guardians, presumably of some education, using such wild words of condemnation ... It is not likely that a medical man, even if young, would undertake something so unpleasant as a post-mortem examination unless he believed that some increase of knowledge might result which would probably benefit his fellow men.[6]

As we have seen in the previous chapter, the issue remains a contemporary concern. In April 2006 the newspaper *USA Today* reported on the stealing of body parts for transplantation to live patients. The article revealed that in the previous nineteen years, 16,800 families were 'represented in lawsuits claiming loved ones' body parts were stolen for profit'.[7] The commotion over the theft (which included the body of celebrated broadcaster Alastair Cook) is echoed in Britain today with the scandals surrounding Professor Dick van Velsen at Alder Hey Hospital and the Bristol babies' hearts. As a result of such examples of public disquiet, the Home Office is currently funding research in Oxford into the non-invasive post-mortem in an effort to allay personal and religious objections to post-mortem.[8]

APPENDIX

Table I. Number of Bodies Received at Provincial Medical Schools 1834–71*

	31 March 1834	1 April 1835
Bath	2	1
Birmingham	10	10
Bristol	4	6
Exeter	5	4
Hull		1
Leeds	4	2
Liverpool	9	6
Manchester	16	10
Newcastle		2
Nottingham	1	1
Sheffield	11	2
TOTAL	62	45
London total:	232 (hospitals); 63 (anatomy schools)	252
Cambridge University:	1	2

*   For all sections of Table I, blank fields indicate that there is no entry in the anatomy records; where the records explicitly state '0', this has been recorded in the data presented here. Furthermore, the anatomy records frequently feature inconsistencies, e.g. in the presentation of the names of cities or individual institutions; anomalies in the data presented here reflect how they appear in the original records.

1833–4:	1833*	1834*
Bath	2	2
Birmingham	23	21
Bristol	17	8
Exeter	1	6
Hull	4	1
Leeds	3	9
Liverpool	6	17
Manchester	13	24

1833–4:	1833*	1834*
Nottingham	1	3
Sheffield	11	20
Warrington	1	1
TOTAL	82	112

*   These figures provide the number of bodies for the whole year. The anatomy records rarely give whole year figures, so this information is something of an anomaly.

1836:	1 January	1 April	31 December
Bath, Walcot Poor House	2	2	1
Birmingham Infirmary			15
Birmingham Workhouse	13	11	
Bristol, General Hospital			2
Bristol Hospital	1	3	
Bristol Infirmary		2	6
Bristol, St Christopher's Parish	3		
Bristol, St Nicholas's Parish	1		
Bristol, St Peter's Hospital	1		4
Exeter	1		
Exeter Workhouse	1		
Hull Infirmary	1		
Hull Workhouse	2		
Leeds House of Recovery	1	1	
Leeds Infirmary	1	1	
Leeds Vagrant Office	1		
Liverpool*		1	
Liverpool Hospital			1
Liverpool Infirmary			2
Liverpool Workhouse	3	3	4
Manchester Coroner			2
Manchester Infirmary	2	5	10
Manchester New Bailey	1		
Manchester Workhouse	3	8	5
Manchester Vagrant Office		1	
Newcastle Coroner			1
Newcastle Upon Tyne (drowned)	1		
Nottingham		1	
Nottingham Workhouse			1
Salisbury		1	
Sheffield Infirmary	1		1
Sheffield Poor House	2	1	3
Stockport			1
Wakefield Coroners			1
Wakefield Prison			1
York Country Hospital			1
TOTAL	42	42	62

1836:	1 January	1 April	31 December
London total:	250	234	200
Hulks:		17	6
Cambridge University:		2	1

*   For 1 April of this year, the original records show an anomaly in presenting data both for 'Liverpool' and for 'Liverpool Workhouse'.

1837:	1 April
Bath, Walcot Poor House	1
Birmingham Infirmary	13
Bristol, General Hospital	2
Bristol Infirmary	2
Bristol, St Peters Hospital	5
Exeter Workhouse	1
Hull Infirmary	1
Hull Vagrant Office	1
Hull Workhouse	1
Leeds House of Recovery	8
Leeds Infirmary	4
Leeds Workhouse	1
Liverpool Workhouse	6
Manchester Coroner	2
Manchester Infirmary	9
Manchester New Bailey Prison	2
Manchester Workhouse	10
Newcastle	1
Norwich Castle	1
Nottingham Workhouse	4
Salisbury	1
Sheffield Poor House	3
TOTAL	79

London total:	335
Hulks:	5
Cambridge University:	2

1838:	1 January	1 April
Bath United Hospital		2
Birmingham Infirmary	10	
Birmingham Workhouse		12
Bristol General		1
Bristol Infirmary	2	4
Bristol, St Peters Hospital	5	1
Exeter Workhouse	1	1
Hull Infirmary	1	1
Hull Lodging House	1	
Hull Vagrant Office	1	
Leeds House of Correction	1	

1838:	1 January	1 April
Leeds House of Recovery		2
Leeds Infirmary	2	1
Leeds Vagrant Office		1
Leeds, Wakefield		2
Liverpool Infirmary	2	1
Liverpool Workhouse	3	3
Manchester Coroner		4
Manchester Infirmary	2	2
Manchester Workhouse	6	3
Newcastle	4	
Salisbury	1	
Sheffield Workhouse	2	
York County Hospital	3	
TOTAL	47	41

London total:	216	310
Hulks:		19
Cambridge University:		2
Oxford University:		1

1839:	1 January	1 April
Birmingham Hospital	1	
Birmingham Infirmary		17
Birmingham, West Bromwich		1
Birmingham Workhouse	10	
Bristol Infirmary	5	18
Bristol General		3
Bristol, St Peters Hospital	3	1
Hull Infirmary	1	2
Hull Gaol		1
Hull Vagrant Office		2
Leeds House of Correction	1	
Leeds House of Recovery		4
Leeds Infirmary		1
Leeds Vagrant Office	2	
Liverpool Hospital	1	2
Liverpool Infirmary	3	2
Liverpool Workhouse		1
Manchester Coroner	1	1
Manchester Infirmary	3	8
Manchester New Bailey Prison	2	
Manchester Workhouse	4	2
Newcastle	2	
Newcastle Coroner	1	1
Newcastle Fever Hospital		2
Nottingham Workhouse		2
Sheffield Infirmary	2	1
Sheffield Workhouse	1	1

1839:	1 January	1 April
York Castle		1
York County Hospital	2	
TOTAL	45	74

London total:	207	189
Hulks:	7	20
Cambridge University:	1	2
Oxford University:		1

1840:	1 January
Bath United Hospital	1
Birmingham Workhouse	16
Bristol General	1
Bristol Infirmary	4
Bristol, St. Peters Hospital	1
Hull Infirmary	1
Hull Vagrant Office	3
Leeds House of Recovery	1
Leeds Infirmary	1
Liverpool Workhouse	3
Manchester Coroner	2
Manchester Infirmary	3
Manchester New Bailey Prison	1
Manchester Workhouse	3 (All bodies to Thomas Turner)
Newcastle Coroner	2
Newcastle, Illegitimate	1
Sheffield Infirmary	2
York House of Correction	1
TOTAL	47

London total:	170
Hulks:	13
Cambridge University:	1

1841:	1 January	1 April
Bath United Hospital	1	
Birmingham Workhouse	9	11
Bristol Infirmary	2	6
Hull Workhouse	3	
Leeds Infirmary	1	2
Leeds Coroner		1
Leeds House of Recovery		2
Leeds Vagrant Office		1

1841:	1 January	1 April
Liverpool Infirmary	1	1
Liverpool Workhouse	3	4
Manchester Coroner		1
Manchester Infirmary	1 (All bodies to Thomas Tuner)	
Manchester New Bailey Prison	1	
Manchester Workhouse	4	5
Newcastle Coroner		1
York Castle		1
Unattributed	2	
St Peters Hospital	6 (Location unspecified – probably Bristol)	
Wakefield House of Correction	2	2
TOTAL	36	38
London total:	222	219
Hulks:	33	40
Cambridge University:	2	1
Oxford University:	1	1
1842:	1 January	1 April
Birmingham Workhouse	12	16
Bristol Infirmary	3	2
Bristol, St Peters Hospital	2	3
Hull Coroner	1	
Hull Infirmary	1	
Hull Vagrant Office		1
Leeds House of Recovery	1	
Leeds Infirmary		2
Liverpool Infirmary	3	2
Liverpool, Northern Hospital	1	
Liverpool Workhouse	1	3
Manchester Infirmary		2
Manchester Workhouse	4 (All bodies to Thomas Tuner)	4 (All bodies to Thomas Turner)
Newcastle, Castle Garth		1
Newcastle Coroner	2	
Newcastle Infirmary	1	2
Nottingham Workhouse	1	
Sheffield Infirmary		1
Wakefield House of Correction	2	
York Hospital	1	
TOTAL	36	39
London total:	159	168
Hulks:	17	
Cambridge University:	1	1 (male)
Oxford University:		1 (male)

1842:*	31 December
Bath	0
Birmingham	5
Bristol	6
Hull	2
Leeds	4
Liverpool	2
Manchester	6
Newcastle	3
Oxford	0
Sheffield	1
York	1
TOTAL	30

* From December 1842 onwards, the anatomy records start to refer simply to city listings and not to specific institutions. In 1859 and 1860 specific institutions are once again listed; however, because these last only for a few entries before reverting back to city listings, they have not been included in the figures below.

Winter Sessions:	1841–2	1842–3
Birmingham	29	19
Bristol	10	11
Cambridge	0	2 (Now in provincial records)
Exeter	0	1
Hull	3	4
Leeds	6	5
Liverpool	10	6
Manchester (Goodlad)	0	3 (46 Mosley Street)
Manchester (Turner)	10	10 (67 Mosley Street)
Newcastle	7	4
Nottingham	1	0
Oxford	0	1 (Now in provincial records)
Sheffield	1	2
York	1	3
TOTAL	78	71

	1842–3	1843–4	1844–5
Bath	0	1	
Birmingham	19	14	18
Bristol	11	6	11
Cambridge	2	1	1
Exeter	1	2	1
Hull	4	3	4
Leeds	5	11	7
Liverpool	6	8	9
Manchester	12 (67 Moseley Street); 4 (46 Mosley Street)	17 (67 Mosley Street); 3 (46 Mosley Street)	17 (67 Mosley Street); 2 (11 Bridge Street)

	1842–3	1843–4	1844–5
Newcastle	5	13	7
Norwich	1	0	
Oxford	1	0	
Sheffield	2	5	7
York	4	0	2
TOTAL	78	84	86

1843:	31 March	30 September	31 December
Bath			1
Birmingham	14		7
Bristol	5		4
Cambridge	2		
Exeter	1		2
Hull	2		2
Leeds	1		3
Liverpool	4		4
Manchester	5 (Turner); 1 (Goodlad)	1	7 (67 Mosley Street); 2 (46 Mosley Street)
Newcastle	1	1	2
Nottingham	0		
Norwich		1	
Oxford	1		
Sheffield	1		3
York	2	1	
TOTAL	40	4	37

1844:	31 March	30 June	30 September	31 December
Birmingham	4	1	2	7
Bristol	2			7
Hull	1			3
Leeds	2	2	4	3
Liverpool	4			1
Manchester	9 (67 Mosley Street); 1 (46 Mosley Street)	1 (67 Mosley Street)		10
Newcastle	7	1	3	2
Sheffield	1	1		4
York				1
TOTAL	31	6	9	38

1845:	30 April	30 June	30 September	31 December
Birmingham	11			9
Bristol	4			5
Exeter	1			

1845:	30 April	30 June	30 September	31 December
Hull	1			1
Leeds	4	1	1	3
Liverpool	8			4
Manchester	1 (11 Bridge Street: Turner? Jordan's house); 8 (67 Mosley Street: Turner)			6
Newcastle	5	2		5
Sheffield	3	1		3
York	1		1	
TOTAL	47	4	2	36

1846:	30 April	30 June	31 December
Birmingham	7		11
Bristol	4		5
Exeter	1		0
Hull	3		1
Leeds	7	1	5
Liverpool	7		5
Manchester	7 (67 Mosley Street); 1 (11 Bridge Street)		4 (67 Mosley Street)
Newcastle	3	1	3
Sheffield	5		1
York	1		0
TOTAL	46	2	35

1847:	30 April	30 June	30 September	31 December
Birmingham	7	1		10
Bristol	6			6
Bury, Lancashire	1			
Exeter	2			0
Hull	2			1
Leeds	11	5		3
Liverpool	6			5
Manchester	12 (67 Mosley Street)			8 (67 Mosley Street)
Newcastle	2			4
Sheffield	5			3
York	1	1	2	2
TOTAL	55	7	2	42

1848:	30 April	30 June	30 September	31 December
Birmingham	9			8
Bristol	1			2

1848:	30 April	30 June	30 September	31 December
Cambridge	2			
Exeter	2			0
Hull	2			0
Leeds	13	3	3	3
Liverpool	7			5
Manchester	5 (67 Mosley Street)			6 (67 Mosley Street)
Newcastle	1			4
Sheffield	2	1		1
York	2			1
TOTAL	46	4	3	30

1849:	30 April	30 June	30 September	31 December
Birmingham	11			3
Bristol	6			1
Cambridge	1 (supplied by a metropolitan source)			
Exeter	0	1		0
Hull	3			1
Leeds	8	2		4
Liverpool	6			4
Manchester	9 (67 Mosley Street); 1 (11 Bridge Street)			6
Newcastle	0	1		3
Sheffield	3			1
York	4		1	1
TOTAL	52	4	1	24

1850:	30 April	30 September	31 December
Birmingham	21		5
Bristol	6		4
Cambridge	1		
Exeter	0	1	
Hull	1		1
Leeds	8	2	5
Liverpool	6		4
Manchester	5 (67 Mosley Street); 1 (11 Bridge Street)	1 (67 Mosley Street)	6 (Mosley Street: Turner); 3 (Chatham Street: Dunville and Southam)
Newcastle	3		3
Sheffield	3	1	5
York	3		
TOTAL	58	5	36

1850–1: Winter and Summer

Birmingham	15
Bristol	9
Cambridge	1
Exeter	2
Hull	2
Leeds	13
Liverpool	11
Manchester	5 (Chatham Street); 11 (Pine Street – previously 67 Mosley Street)
Newcastle	6
Sheffield	8
York	1
TOTAL	84

1851:	1 January–30 April	30 April–30 June	30 September	31 December
Birmingham	10			10 (Queens); 1 (Sydenham)
Bristol	5			3
Cambridge		1		
Exeter	2			1
Hull	1			0
Leeds	6	1	1	8
Liverpool	7			4
Manchester	3 (Pine Street); 2 (Chatham Street)	1 (Pine Street)		7 (Pine Street); 4 (Chatham Street); 1 (Bridge Street)
Newcastle	3			5 (Newcastle School); 3 (Newcastle College)
Sheffield	3			4
York	1			1
TOTAL	43	3	1	52

1852:	1 January–30 April	30 April–30 June	30 September	31 December
Birmingham	11 (Queens); 2 (Sydenham)			9 (Queens); 3 (Sydenham)
Bristol	7			5
Cambridge		1		
Exeter	0			1
Hull	2	1		1
Leeds	9	2	1	5
Liverpool	10			5

1852:	1 January–30 April	30 April–30 June	30 September	31 December
Manchester	10 (Pine Street); 4 (Chatham Street); 1 (Bridge Street)	2 (Pine Street); 1 (Chatham Street)		11 (Pine Street); 6 (Chatham Street)
Newcastle	1	2	2	7
Sheffield	2			1
York	2			1
TOTAL	61	9	3	55

1853:	1 January–30 April	May–June	30 September	31 December
Birmingham	7 (Queens); 2 (Sydenham)			11
Bristol	5			5
Cambridge		1		
Exeter	2			
Hull	2			
Leeds	9		1	7
Liverpool	10			6
Manchester	10 (Pine Street); 7 (Chatham Street)			7 (Chatham Street); 8 (Pine Street)
Newcastle	2	2		5
Sheffield	2			5
York	1			
TOTAL	59	3	1	54

Submitted to the President of Royal College of Surgeons: Number of Bodies to Provincial Anatomy Schools, Winter and Summer 1850–1

1850-1:	Winter	Summer	Total
Birmingham	15	0	15
Bristol	9	0	9
Cambridge	0	1	1
Exeter	2	0	2
Hull	2	0	2
Leeds	11	2	13
Liverpool	11	0	11
Manchester	5 (Chatham Street); 9 (Pine Street)	0 (Chatham Street); 2 (Pine Street)	5 (Chatham Street); 11 (Pine Street)
Newcastle	6	0	6
Sheffield	8	0	8
York	1	0	1
TOTAL	79	5	84

Return Submitted to Court of Examiners, Royal College of Surgeons, 21 June 1853

	Winter 1851–2	Summer 1851–2	Total 1851–2	Winter 1852–3	Summer 1852–3	Total 1852–3
Birmingham	21 (Queens); 3 (Sydenham)	0	21 (Queens); 3 (Sydenham)	16 (Queens); 5 (Sydenham)	0 (Queens); 0 (Sydenham)	16 (Queens); 5 (Sydenham)
Bristol	10	0	10	10	0	10
Cambridge	0	1	1	0	1	1
Exeter	1	0	1	3	0	3
Hull	2	1	3	3	0	3
Leeds	17	3	20	14	0	14
Liverpool	14	0	14	12	0	12
Manchester	2 (Bridge Street); 8 (Chatham Street); 17 (Pine Street)	0 (Bridge Street); 1 (Chatham Street); 2 (Pine Street)	2 (Bridge Street); 9 (Chatham Street); 19 (Pine Street)	0 (Bridge Street); 13 (Chatham Street); 21 (Pine Street)	0 (Bridge Street); 0 (Chatham Street); 0 (Pine Street)	0 (Bridge Street); 13 (Chatham Street); 21 (Pine Street)
Newcastle	9	4	13	9	2	11
Sheffield	6	0	6	3	0	3
York	3	0	3	2	0	2
TOTAL	113	12	125	111	3	114

1854:	1 January–30 April	30 April–30 June	30 September
Birmingham	6	1	
Bristol	3		
Cambridge	1		
Exeter	2		
Hull	2		
Leeds	8		3
Liverpool	5		
Manchester	11 (Pine Street); 9 (Chatham Street)	1 (Pine Street)	1
Newcastle	5	3	1
Sheffield	2		
York	2	2	1
TOTAL	56	7	6

1855:	30 April	30 June	30 September	31 December
Birmingham	12			13
Bristol	4			5
Cambridge				1
Exeter				1
Hull	4	1		2
Leeds	9	1		5
Liverpool	6			5

1855:	30 April	30 June	30 September	31 December
Manchester	9 (Pine Street); 9 (Chatham Street)	1 (Pine Street); 1 (Chatham Street)	2 (Bridge Street)	7 (Chatham Street); 6 (Pine Street); 1 (Bridge Street)
Newcastle	6	3		4
Sheffield	2			2
York	2			2
TOTAL	63	7	2	54

1856:	31 March	30 June	31 December
Birmingham	12		14
Bristol	4	1	5
Cambridge		1	
Exeter			1
Hull	2		2
Leeds	6	3	6
Liverpool	7	1	7
Manchester	5 (Chatham Street); 6 (Pine Street)	1 (Bridge Street); 2 (Chatham Strret)	12
Newcastle	6	4	4
Sheffield	2		1
York	1	1	1
TOTAL	51	14	53

1857:	31 March	30 June	31 December
Birmingham	12		15
Bristol	3		5
Cambridge			1
Exeter	1		0
Hull	2		0
Leeds	3	6	7
Liverpool	7	1	8
Manchester	17	1 (Bridge Street)	4
Newcastle	6	2	5
Sheffield	4		3
York	2		5
TOTAL	57	10	53

1858:	31 March	30 June	30 September	31 December
Birmingham	2			13
Bristol	5	1		4
Cambridge				2
Exeter	0			0
Hull	5			3
Leeds	2	7	2	4
Liverpool	7	1	2	6
Manchester	10		1	14

1858:	31 March	30 June	30 September	31 December
Newcastle	6	2		6
Sheffield	1			3
York	0			2
TOTAL	38	11	5	57

1859:	31 March	30 June	31 December	
Bath				
Birmingham	9		12	
Bristol	7	1	6	
Cambridge	1	1	0	
Exeter	0		0	
Hull	4		1	
Leeds	6	4	2	
Liverpool	7		9	
Manchester	12		6	
Newcastle	7	3	3	
Sheffield	1		4	
York	1		0	
TOTAL	55	9	43	

1860:	31 March	30 June	30 September	31 December
Bath	1			
Birmingham	10			6
Bristol	9			5
Cambridge		1		1
Exeter	0			0
Hull	2			4
Leeds	11	2	1	3
Liverpool	11			9
Manchester	23		1	15
Newcastle	10	2		8
Sheffield	1		1	5
York	0			0
TOTAL	78	5	3	56

1861:	31 March	30 June	30 September	31 December
Bath	1			
Birmingham	7	1		8
Bristol	5			4
Cambridge		1		1
Hull	3			3
Leeds	8	3	2	7
Liverpool	14	2		7
Manchester	13			9
Newcastle	5			6
Sheffield	5			4
TOTAL	61	7	2	49

1862:	31 March	30 June	31 December	
Bath	0	0	0	
Birmingham	8	2	10	
Bristol	5	0	5	
Cambridge	2		2	
Hull	1	1	3	
Leeds	6	3	6	
Liverpool	14	1	9	
Manchester	13	3	10	
Newcastle	4	1	8	
Sheffield	4	0	4	
TOTAL	57	11	57	

1863:	31 March	30 June	30 September	31 December
Bath	0			0
Birmingham	8			8
Bristol	4			4
Cambridge	1			
Hull	2	1	1	3
Leeds	4	1	3	4
Liverpool	12		1	9
Manchester	8	1	1	2
Newcastle	4	1	1	7
Sheffield	3	1		3
TOTAL	46	5	7	40

1864:	31 March	30 June	30 September	31 December
Bath	0			1
Birmingham	10			5
Bristol	4			3
Cambridge	2			2
Hull	3			1
Leeds	13	3	3	7
Liverpool	12			11
Manchester	16			16
Newcastle	3	2		7
Oxford University				1
Sheffield	3			3
TOTAL	66	5	3	57

1865:	31 March	30 June	30 September	31 December
Bath	0			0
Birmingham	13			6
Bristol	3	2		2
Cambridge	2			2
Hull	1			1
Leeds	6	3	1	10
Liverpool	12	4		10

1865:	31 March	30 June	30 September	31 December
Manchester	14			16
Newcastle	4	2		4
Sheffield	4			1
TOTAL	59	11	1	52

1866:	31 March	30 June	31 December
Bath	0		0
Birmingham	7	2	8
Bristol	7		3
Cambridge	4		3
Hull	1	1	3
Leeds	6	3	10
Liverpool	16	1	15
Manchester	1		16
Newcastle	2	2	6
Sheffield	5		4
TOTAL	61	9	68

1867:	31 March	30 June	31 December
Bath	0		
Birmingham	10		12
Bristol	5		2
Cambridge	2	1	1
Hull	3		4
Leeds	6	1	6
Liverpool	16	1	9
Manchester	18	1	6
Newcastle	4		5
Salford Royal Hospital			1
Sheffield	5	1	6
TOTAL	69	5	52

1868:	31 March	30 June	30 September	31 December
Birmingham	7			8
Bristol	5			5
Cambridge	2		1	3
Hull	2			0
Leeds	6	2	1	9
Liverpool	16		1	10
Manchester	21			14
Newcastle	4	1		3
Sheffield	3			4
TOTAL	66	3	3	56

1869:	31 March	30 June	30 September	31 December
Birmingham	13	3		14
Bristol	5			5
Cambridge	5			5
Hull	1		2	0
Leeds	5		1	5
Liverpool	16	1	1	8
Manchester	15			21
Newcastle	4	1		5
Sheffield	5	1		1
Wakefield			1	
TOTAL	69	6	5	64

1870:	31 March	30 June	30 September	31 December
Birmingham	5	1	2	13
Bristol	4			4
Cambridge	1		1	1
Hull	0			0
Leeds	6	2	1	11
Liverpool	12	3	2	11
Manchester	22			20
Newcastle	4		1	6
Sheffield	4	1		4
TOTAL	58	7	7	70

1871:	31 March	30 June
Birmingham	12	1
Bristol	4	1
Cambridge	5	1
Hull	0	0
Leeds	2	6
Liverpool	11	0
Manchester	16	1
Newcastle	5	1
Sheffield	4	1
TOTAL	59	12

Source: Compiled from Anatomy Inspectorate returns, NA, MH 74/10, MH 74/11, MH 74/12, MH 74/13, MH 74/14, MH 74/15, MH 74/16, MH 74/36, MH 74/37, MH 74/38.

Table II. Number of Pupils at the Provincial Schools of Anatomy 1853–63*

	53–4	54–5	55–6	56–7	57–8†	58–9	59–60	60–1	61–2	62–3	63–4	64–5
B'ham Queens	47	40	58	53		54	13	37	32	45	25	24
B'ham Sydenham						32	40	42	36	18	31	51
Bristol	35		21	24		25	18	13	17	19	18	26
Cambridge	0		0	0		0	0	0	13	0	0	0
Durham	24		24	17		54	51	50				
Exeter	9		0	0		0	0	0	0	0	0	0
Hull	11		11	15		13	20	18	14	18	13	8
Leeds	35		40	37		35	36	40	32	23	30	28
Liverpool	31		0	0		24	23	33	24	22	17	20
M'cr Pine	69								51‡	59‡	45‡	42‡
M'cr Chatham	55	55	54	87		70	77	70				
Newcastle	24		34	29					41	28	27	38
Sheffield	13		9			12	10	13	11	16	8	10
York	11		11	12		12	0	0	0	0	0	0
Total	364	95	262	274		331	288	316	271	248	214	247

*   Blank fields indicate that there is no entry in the records; where the records explicitly state '0', this has been recorded in the data presented here.

†   There is no data for the year 1857–8 due to inconsistency in the record-keeping.

‡   For the years 1860–1 to 1864–5 the numbers indicate the combined total of students for Manchester.

Source: NA, MH 74/10.

Table III. Oxford Bodies 1894–1914

Botley Cemetery

Total burials	468
Museum	182
Reading	79
Leicester	46
Manchester	7
Witney	2
Camberwell	1

Source: OCA/C/ENG/1/A1/2.

Wolvercote Cemetery

Reading	18
Manchester	6
London Country Asylum	1
Witney	1

Source: OCA/C/ENG/1/A10/2.

Rose Hill Cemetery

Reading	7
Whitechapel	1
Witney	2

Source: OCA/C/ENG/1/A7/1.

Table IV. Death and Post-Mortem Rates at the Radcliffe Infirmary 1845–99

	Deaths	Post-Mortems	Handwritten Notes
1845	17	–	
1846	21	10	
1847	54	32	
1848	39	22	
1849	46	27	
1850	35	21	
1851	32	9	
1852	31	0	
1853	34	10	
1854	33	6	
1855	38	17	
1856	25	5	
1857	17	5	
1858	42	0	
1859	26	1	
1860	28	1	no pm 2x
1861	32	0	no pm 3x
1862	32	0	no pm 1x
1863	32	0	no pm 1x
1864	43	0	
1865	36	0	
1866	33	0	
1867	52	2	
1868	25	0	
1869	54	0	
1870	57	22	no pm 2x, 1 refused
1871	54	12	
1872	60	0	no pm 2x
1873	45	0	no pm 2x
1874	–	–	
1875	–	–	
1876	–	–	
1877	–	–	
1878	48	8	no pm 3x
1879	30	10	no pm 5x
1880	60	24	No pm 5x, 3 'not allowed'
1881	53	32	1 pm 'refused'
1882	54	39	1 pm 'refused'
1883	55	31	
1884	65	35	
1885	85	32	7 coroners' inquests
1886	67	48	
1887	83	66	

1888	64	33
1889	77	32
1890	55	25
1891	67	44
1892	84	42
1893	70	29
1894	78	38
1895	89	24
1896	92	51
1897	110	19
1898	77	28
1899	96	2

Source: Death Registers, RI 9 B/1/1–5.

NOTES

Introduction

1. R. Richardson, *Death, Dissection and the Destitute* (London: Penguin, 1989).
2. T. Marshall, *Murdering to Dissect: Grave-Robbing, Frankenstein and the Anatomy Literature* (Manchester: Manchester University Press, 1995), p. 330.
3. R. L. Blakely and J. M. Harrington (eds), *Bones in the Basement: Post-Mortem Racism in Nineteenth-Century Medical Training* (Washington, DC and London: Smithsonian Institution, 1997); D. G. Lawrence, 'Resurrection and Legislation on Body-Snatching in Relation to the Anatomy Act in the Province of Quebec', *Bulletin of the History of Medicine,* 32 (1958), pp 408–24; R. MacGillivray, 'Body-Snatching in Ontario', *Canadian Bulletin of Medical History*, 5 (1988), pp. 51–60; M. Sappol, *A Traffic of Dead Bodies: Anatomy and Embodied Social Identity in Nineteenth-Century America* (Princeton, NJ and Woodstock: Princeton University Press, 2002); S. M. Shultz, *Body Snatching: The Robbing of Graves for the Education of Physicians in Early Nineteenth-Century America* (Jefferson, NC and London: McFarland and Co., 1992).
4. H. MacDonald, *Possessing the Dead: The Artful Science of Anatomy* (Melbourne: Melbourne University Press, 2010).
5. M. E. Fissell, *Patients, Power and the Poor in Eighteenth-Century Bristol* (Cambridge: Cambridge University Press, 1991); E. Hurren, 'A Pauper Dead-House: The Expansion of the Cambridge Anatomical Teaching School under the Late-Victorian Poor Law, 1870–1914', *Medical History*, 48 (2004), pp. 69–94; E. Knox, 'The Body Politic: Body-Snatching, the Anatomy Act and the Poor on Tyneside', *North East Labour History Society Bulletin*, 24 (1990), pp. 19–34.
6. P. Linebaugh, 'The Tyburn Riot against the Surgeons', in D. Hay, P. Linebaugh, J. Rule and E. P. Thompson (eds), *Albion's Fatal Tree: Crime and Society in Eighteenth-Century England* (Harmondsworth: Penguin, 1975), pp. 65–117, on p. 109.
7. Anatomy lecturer at the Company of Surgeons, 1783; demonstrator in anatomy at St Thomas's Hospital, and surgeon at Guy's Hospital, 1800; surgeon to George IV, 1820.
8. G. Rudé, *The Crowd in History: A Study of Popular Disturbances in France and England 1730–1848* (London: Serif, 1998), p. 267.
9. S. Burrell and G. Gill, 'The Liverpool Cholera Epidemic of 1832 and Anatomical Mistrust and Civil Unrest', *Journal of the History of Medicine and Allied Sciences*, 60 (2005), pp. 478–98.

10. F. K. Donnelly, 'The Destruction of the Sheffield School of Anatomy in 1835: A Popular Response to Class Legislation', *Transactions of the Hunter Archaeological Society*, 10 (1975), pp. 167–72.
11. R. C. Maulitz, *Morbid Appearances: The Anatomy of Pathology in the Early Nineteenth Century* (Cambridge: Cambridge University Press, 1987), p. 150.
12. E. Hurren, 'Labourers are Revolting: Penalising the Poor and a Political Reaction in the Brixworth Union, Northamptonshire, 1875–1885', *Rural History*, 11 (2000), pp. 37–55.
13. M. Weatherall, *Gentlemen, Scientists and Doctors: Medicine at Cambridge 1800–1940* (Woodbridge: Boydell Press and Cambridge University Library, 2000), p. 219.
14. Hurren, 'A Pauper Dead-House'.
15. This argument is echoed effectively by L. H. Lees, *The Solidarities of Strangers: The English Poor Laws and the People, 1700–1948* (Cambridge: Cambridge University Press, 1998).
16. J. V. Pickstone, 'Ferriar's Fever to Kay's Cholera: Disease and Social Structure in Cottonopolis', *History of Science*, 22 (1984), pp. 400–19, on p. 414.
17. R. Porter, *Bodies Politic: Disease, Death and Doctors in Britain, 1650–1901* (London: Reaktion Books, 2001), p. 240.
18. R. Quinault and J. Stevenson (eds), *Popular Protest and Public Order: Six Studies in British History 1790–1920* (London: Allen and Unwin, 1974), p. 28. See also J. E. Archer, *Social Unrest and Popular Protest in England 1780–1840* (Cambridge: Cambridge University Press, 2000), p. 4.
19. F. Engels, *The Condition of the Working Class in England* (St Albans: Granada, 1982), p. 316.
20. J. Rugg, 'The Origins and Progress of Cemetery Establishment in Britain', in P. C. Jupp and G. Howarth (eds), *The Changing Face of Death: Historical Accounts of Death and Disposal* (London: Macmillan, 1997), pp. 105–19, on p. 116.
21. The Apothecaries Act of 1815 required surgeon-apothecaries desiring the LSA qualification to undergo five years of apprenticeship and courses in medicine and surgery.
22. J. V. Pickstone, *Medicine and Industrial Society: A History of Hospital Development in Manchester and its Region 1752–1946* (Manchester: Manchester University Press, 1985), p. 48.
23. S. C. Lawrence, 'Anatomy and Address: Creating Medical Gentlemen in Eighteenth-Century London', in V. Nutton and R. Porter (eds), *The History of Medical Education in Britain* (Amsterdam and Atlanta, GA: Editions Rodopi BV, 1995), pp. 199–228.
24. C. Lawrence, *Medical Theory, Surgical Practice* (London and New York: Routledge, 1992), p. 31.
25. Sappol, *A Traffic of Dead Bodies*, p. 60.
26. J. Bellers, *An Essay Towards the Improvement of Physick in Twelve Proposals by which the Lives of Many Thousands of the Rich as well as of the Poor may be Saved Yearly* (London: J. Sowle, 1714).
27. Fissell, *Patients, Power and the Poor*, pp. 199–200.
28. Ibid., p. 162.
29. H. MacDonald, *Human Remains: Dissection and its Histories* (New Haven, CT: Yale University Press, 2005), p. 141.
30. Ibid., p. 195.
31. MacDonald, *Possessing the Dead*, ch. 5.

1 Medical Education in Oxford and Manchester before the 1832 Anatomy Act

1. K. Park, 'The Criminal and the Saintly Body: Autopsy and Dissection in Renaissance Italy', *Renaissance Quarterly*, 47 (1994), pp. 1–33, on p. 4. See also G. Ferrari, 'Public Anatomy Lessons and the Carnival: The Anatomy Theatre of Bologna', *Past and Present*, 117 (1987), pp. 50–106.
2. Park, 'The Criminal and the Saintly Body', p. 14.
3. L. S. King and M. C. Meehan, 'A History of the Autopsy', *American Journal of Pathology*, 73 (1973), pp. 514–44.
4. Quoted in I. Loudon, 'Medical Education and Medical Reform', in V. Nutton and R. Porter (eds), *The History of Medical Education in Britain* (Amsterdam and Atlanta, GA: Editions Rodopi BV, 1995), pp. 229–49, on p. 232.
5. T. Gelfand, 'The "Paris Manner" of Dissection: Student Anatomical Dissection in Early Eighteenth-Century Paris', *Bulletin of the History of Medicine*, 46 (1972), pp. 99–130.
6. J. G. Crosse, *Sketches of Medical Schools of Paris* (London: J Callow, 1815), p. 49.
7. C. Lawrence, 'Incommunicable Knowledge: Science, Technology and the Clinical Art in Britain 1850–1914', *Journal of Contemporary History*, 20 (1985), pp. 503–20, on p. 506.
8. Select Committee on Medical Education, 1834, quoted in Richardson, *Death, Dissection and the Destitute*, p. 34.
9. A. Digby, *Making a Medical Living: Doctors and Patients in the English Market for Medicine, 1720–1911* (Cambridge: Cambridge University Press, 1994), p. 54.
10. T. N. Bonner, *Becoming a Physician: Medical Education in Britain, France, Germany, and the United States, 1750–1945* (Oxford and New York: Oxford University Press, 1995), p. 101.
11. Digby, *Making a Medical Living*, p. 91.
12. L. Rosner, *Medical Education in the Age of Improvement* (Edinburgh: Edinburgh University Press, 1991), p. 47.
13. C. Lawrence, 'Alexander Monro Primus and the Edinburgh Manner of Anatomy', *Bulletin of the History of Medicine*, 62 (1988), pp. 193–214, on p. 195.
14. J. H. Green, *The Touchstone of Medical Reform Addressed to Sir Robert Harry Inglis Bart MP* (London: Samuel Highley, 1841), p. 16.
15. W. Moore, *The Knife Man: The Extraordinary Life and Times of John Hunter, Father of Modern Surgery* (London: Transworld Publishers, 2005), p. 122.
16. *The Diary of Richard Kay 1716–51 of Baldingstone, near Bury: A Lancashire Doctor*, ed. W. Brockbank and F. Kenworthy (Manchester: Chetham Society, 1968).
17. Evidence of Sir Astley Cooper to the Select Committee on Medical Education, quoted in P. Stanley, *For Fear of Pain: British Surgery 1790–1850* (Amsterdam and New York: Editions Rodopi BV, 2003), p. 30.
18. J. Bell, *Letters on Professional Character and Manners: On the Education of a Surgeon and the Duties and Qualifications of a Physician* (Edinburgh: J Moir, 1810), p. 579.
19. Digby, *Making a Medical Living*, p. 54.
20. Ibid., p. 196.
21. A. Guerrini, 'Anatomists and Entrepreneurs in Early Eighteenth-Century London', *Journal of the History of Medicine and Allied Sciences*, 59 (2004), pp. 219–39, on p. 221.
22. W. Hunter, *Two Introductory Lectures, Delivered by Dr William Hunter, for his Last Course of Anatomical Lectures at his Theatre in Windmill-Street* (London: J. Johnson, 1784), p. 88.

23. G. C. Peachey, *A Memoir of William and John Hunter* (Plymouth: Brendon, 1924), p. 80.

24. R. Campbell, *The London Tradesman* (Newton Abbott: David and Charles, 1969), p. 44.

25. J. Gregory, *Lectures on the Duties and Qualifications of a Physician* (London: W. Stahan and T. Cadell, 1773), pp. 5–6.

26. R. Davies, *Epistle to the Reverend Dr Hales on the General State of Education in the Universities with a Particular View to the Philosophic and Medical Education, being Introductory to Essays on the Blood* (Bath: M. Cooper, 1759), p. 4.

27. E. Harrison, *Remarks on the Ineffective State of the Practice of Physic in Great Britain, with Proposals for its Future Regulation and Improvement* (London: R. Bickerstaff, 1806), pp. 1 and 4.

28. T. Alcock, 'An Essay on the Education and Duties of the General Practitioner in Medicine and Surgery', *Transactions of the Associated Apothecaries and Apothecary-Surgeons* (1823), pp. 1–135, on pp. 1, 96 and 73.

29. T. Beddoes, *A Letter to the Right Honourable Sir Joseph Banks on the Causes and Removal of the Prevailing Discontents, Imperfections and Abuses in Medicine* (London: Richard Phillips, 1808).

30. W. Chamberlaine, *Tirocinium Medicum; or a Dissertation on the Duties of Youth Apprenticed to the Medical Profession* (London: privately printed, 1812), p. 65.

31. T. Turner, *Outlines of a System of Medico-Chirurgical Education Containing Illustrations of the Application of Anatomy, Physiology and Other Sciences to the Principal Practical Points in Medicine and Surgery* (Manchester: Underwood, 1824), p. 6.

32. J. Parkinson, *The Hospital Pupil; or an Essay Intended to Facilitate the Study of Medicine and Surgery in Four Letters* (London: H. D. Symonds, 1800), p. 76.

33. *London Medical Gazette*, 1 (8 December 1827), p. 10.

34. T. S. Smith, 'The Uses of the Dead to the Living', *Westminster Review*, 2 (1824), pp. 59–94, on p. 80; Thomas Southwood Smith was physician to the London Fever Hospital and in 1839 founded the Health of Towns Association; he is famed for dissecting the body of Jeremy Bentham.

35. Ibid., pp. 59–60.

36. Papers from the Select Committee on Anatomy (hereafter SCA), Evidence of Astley Cooper, 1828, vol. 7, Part 1, p. 15.

37. Surgeon to Westminster Hospital, 1827–43; president of the Royal College of Surgeons, 1833, 1841 and 1854; Royal College of Surgeons professor of anatomy and surgery, 1823–31.

38. G. Guthrie, *A Letter to the Right Honorable the Secretary of State for the Home Department Containing Remarks on the Report of the Select Committee of the House of Commons on Anatomy* (London: W. Sams, 1829), pp. 3–4.

39. *Medico-Chirurgical Review*, 12 (1830), pp. 95–6.

40. T. Turner, *A Practical Treatise on the Arterial System* (London: Longman, 1825), p. 193.

41. *Edinburgh Medical and Surgical Journal*, 26 (1809), pp. 67–72, on pp. 67 and 71.

42. 'Observations of Medical Reform by a Member of the University of Oxford', *Pamphleteer*, 2 (1814), pp. 414–31, on p. 414.

43. J. Farre, *An Apology for British Anatomy, and an Incitement to the Study of Morbid Anatomy* (London: Longman, 1827), p. 5.

44. J. Mann, *Recollections of my Early and Professional Life* (London: W. Rider and Sons, 1887), pp. 95–6.

45. Physician to Meath Hospital, 1821–43; president of King and Queen's College of Physicians of Ireland, 1843–4.
46. R. J. Graves, 'On Clinical Instruction', *London Medical Gazette*, 10 (1832), pp. 402–3.
47. 'Medical Education in England', *London Medical Gazette* (8 December 1827), p. 10.
48. Editor of *Lancet* from 1823; MP for Finsbury, 1835–52; coroner for West Middlesex, 1839.
49. *Lancet*, 1 (19 October 1823), p. 98.
50. *Lancet*, 2 (1830–2), pp. 669–70.
51. Hunter, *Two Introductory Lectures*, p. 73.
52. Bellers, *An Essay Towards the Improvement of Physick in Twelve Proposals*, p. 6.
53. Ibid., p. 7.
54. Educated at Edinburgh and Leiden; settled in Manchester, 1767; founder of the Manchester Literary and Philosophical Society.
55. J. Aiken, *Thoughts on Hospitals: With a Letter to the Author by Thomas Percival* (London: Joseph Jackson, 1771), pp. 86–7.
56. S. C. Lawrence, *Charitable Knowledge: Hospital Pupils and Practitioners in Eighteenth-Century London* (Cambridge: Cambridge University Press, 1996), p. 72.
57. W. F. Bynum, *Science and the Practice of Medicine in the Nineteenth Century* (Cambridge: Cambridge University Press, 1994), p. 28.
58. Lawrence, *Charitable Knowledge*, p. 108.
59. M. Durey, *The Return of the Plague: British Society and the Cholera 1831–2* (Dublin: Gill and Macmillan, 1979), p. 108.
60. Letter dated 24 June 1664, in R. Boyle, *Works*, 14 vols (London: W. Johnston, 1772), vol. 4, pp. 468–70.
61. Letter dated 4 June 1663, in ibid., p. 467.
62. Letter dated 24 June 1664, in ibid., pp. 471–2.
63. W. H. Quarrell and W. J. C. Quarrell, *Oxford in 1710 from the Travels of Zacharias Conrad von Uffenbach* (Oxford: Basil Blackwell, 1928), pp. 36–7.
64. Lee's Reader in Anatomy, 1816–45; Regius Professor of Medicine, 1822–51.
65. E. G. W. Bill, *Education at Christ Church, Oxford, 1660–1800* (Oxford: Clarendon Press, 1988), p. 318.
66. H. M. Sinclair and A. H. T. Robb-Smith, *A Short History of Anatomical Teaching in Oxford* (Oxford: Oxford University Press, 1950), p. 38.
67. Corpus Christi College, MS.263 fol. 128, Diary of Bryan Twynne. Twynne was admitted as a scholar at Corpus Christi in 1594 at the age of eighteen. He was fellow of Corpus 1605; MA 1603; BD 1610; reader 1614; and died in 1644.
68. A. Muehry, *Observations on the Comparative State of Medicine in France, England and Germany during a Journey into these Countries in the Year 1835* (Philadelphia, PA: A. Waldie, 1838), p. 77.
69. C. G. Carus, *The King of Saxony's Journey through England and Scotland in the Year 1844* (London: Chapman and Hall, 1846), p. 186.
70. Ibid., p. 188.
71. H. W. Acland, *Oxford and Modern Medicine, a Letter to Dr James Andrew* (Oxford and London: Henry Frowde, 1890), p. 12.
72. H. D. Rolleston, 'The History of Clinical Medicine (Principally of Clinical Teaching) in the British Isles', *Proceedings of the Royal Society of Medicine*, 32 (1939), pp. 1185–90, on p. 1189.

73. Aldrichian Professor of Medicine, 1824–57; Lichfield Professor Clinical Medicine, 1830–57; Regius Professor, 1851–7; physician to Radcliffe Infirmary, 1824–57; Fellow of the Royal College of Physicians, 1822.

74. A. H. T. Robb-Smith, 'Medical Education', in M. G. Brock and M. C. Curthoys (eds), *The History of the University of Oxford, Volume VI: Nineteenth-Century Oxford, Part 1* (Oxford: Clarendon Press, 2000), pp. 563–82, on p. 570.

75. Select Committee on Medical Education, 1834, Q4468.

76. Rosner, *Medical Education in the Age of Improvement*, p. 23.

77. Lee's Reader in Anatomy at Oxford 1845, Regius and Clinical Professor Medicine 1857. Acland's career is covered extensively in Chapters 4 and 5.

78. Member of the Royal College of Surgeons, 1805; senior surgeon at St George's, 1822–40; King's Personal Surgeon, 1828, and Sergeant-Surgeon under William IV and Victoria; president of the Royal College of Surgeons, 1844; president of the General Medical Council, 1858.

79. J. B. Atlay, *Sir Henry Wentworth Acland, Bart, KCB, FRS, Regius Professor of Medicine in the University of Oxford. A Memoir* (London: Smith, Elder and Co., 1903), p. 33.

80. Ibid., p. 122.

81. L. Stone, *The University in Society*, 2 vols (Princeton, NJ: Princeton University Press, 1975), vol. 1, p. 37.

82. 'A Vindication of the London College of Physicians', *Lancet*, 1 (1827–8), pp. 757–8.

83. Stone, *The University in Society*, vol. 1, p. 61.

84. 'Observations on Medical Reform by a Member of the University of Oxford', *Pamphleteer*, 2 (1814), pp. 414–31, on p. 423.

85. R. M. Kerrison, *An Inquiry into the Present State of the Medical Profession in England* (London: Longman and Co., 1814), p. 17.

86. 'A Vindication of Scottish Graduates', *Lancet*, 1 (1827–8), pp. 759–62, on p. 761.

87. Radcliffe Infirmary, RI C/I/9, Board of Governors Minutes, 27 February 1839.

88. S. Hallifax, *A Sermon for the Governors of Addenbrooke's Hospital* (Cambridge: J. Archdeacon, 1771), p. 11.

89. J. G. Adami, *Charles White of Manchester (1728–1813) and the Arrest of Puerperal Fever* (London: Hodder and Stoughton, 1922). White, known as an obstetrician, was apprenticed to his father and attended the Hunters' London lectures and medical lectures in Edinburgh; he founded Manchester Infirmary in 1755, and was chief surgeon for thirty-eight years.

90. W. J. Elwood and A. F. Tuxford, *Some Manchester Doctors* (Manchester: Manchester University Press, 1984), p. 67.

91. T. Turner, *Memoir of Thomas Turner Esq. FRCS FLS, by a Relative with an Introduction by the Rev. David Bell* (London: Simpkin, Marshall and Co., 1875), p. 27.

92. F. Nicholson, 'The Literary and Philosophical Society 1781–1851', *Memoirs of the Manchester Literary and Philosophical Society*, 68 (1924), pp. 97–148, on p. 147.

93. A. Thackray, 'Natural Knowledge in a Cultural Context: The Manchester Model', *American Historical Review*, 79 (1974), pp. 672–701, on p. 678.

94. T. Barnes, 'Proposals for Establishing in Manchester a Plan of Liberal Education, for Young Men Designed for Civil and Active Life Whether in Trade, or in Any of the Professions', *Manchester Memoirs*, 2 (1785), pp. 30–5, on p. 35.

95. *Manchester Guardian*, 5 October 1836.

96. Elwood and Tuxford, *Some Manchester Doctors*, p. 70.

97. Ibid., p. 71.

98. T. Turner, *An Address to the Inhabitants of Lancashire and of the Adjoining Counties on the Present State of the Medical Profession with Remarks on the Elementary Education of the Student, and the Best Means of its Acquirement. Intended to Shew the Practicality and Importance of Establishing a School (on a More Extended Scale) in Manchester for the Cultivation of Medical and Surgical Knowledge* (London: Longman; Manchester: Underwood, 1825), p. 7.

99. Ibid., pp. 17–19.

100. *Memoir of Thomas Turner*, p. 86.

101. S. T. Anning, 'Provincial Medical Schools in the Nineteenth Century', in F. N. L. Poynter (ed.), *The Evolution of Medical Education in Britain* (London: Pitman, 1966), pp. 121–34, on p. 121.

102. W. Brockbank, *The Foundation of Provincial Medical Education in England and of the Manchester School in Particular* (Manchester: Manchester University Press, 1936), p. 89.

103. S. V. F. Butler, 'Science and the Education of Doctors in the Nineteenth Century: A Study of British Medical Schools with Particular Reference to the Uses and Development of Physiology', (PhD thesis, University of Manchester Institute of Science and Technology, 1982).

104. University of Manchester, John Rylands Library (hereafter MUJRL), Manchester Medical Collection – biographical files (hereafter MMC), 6 October 1826.

105. *London Medical Gazette* (16 February 1828).

106. Brockbank, *Foundation of Provincial Medical Education in England*, p. 97.

107. Manchester Royal Infirmary (hereafter MRI), Minutes of Special Medical Committee 1822–47.

108. MUJRL, MMC, letter, 18 February 1831.

109. MUJRL, MMC, 8 November 1830, 14 March 1831.

110. MRI, Minutes of Special Medical Committee 1822–47, 14 March 1831.

111. Ibid., 2 April 1832.

112. MRI, Minutes of Weekly Board of Governors 1843–5, 28 June 1845, vol. 24.

113. Lecturer in pathology at Jordan's school, 1825; man-midwife to Lying-In Charity, 1829; founder of Marsden Street Anatomy School; honorary surgeon to Manchester Royal Infirmary, 1837.

114. MRI, Minutes of Manchester Infirmary 1818, p. 153; and Manchester Medical Collection, biographical files, MMC/2/Fawdington.

115. MRI, Minutes of Manchester Infirmary 1818, p. 30.

2 Dissection in Oxford and Manchester: Supply and Demand before 1832

1. T. Hearne, *Remarks and Collections*, 11 vols (Oxford: Oxford University Press, 1885–1921).

2. V. A. C. Gatrell provides extensive data on capital convictions and executions in the eighteenth and nineteenth centuries, most detailed for London, in *The Hanging Tree: Execution and the English People 1770–1868* (Oxford: Oxford University Press, 1994), appendix 2.

3. J. M. Ball, *The Sack-'em-up Men: An Account of the Rise and Fall of the Modern Resurrectionists* (London: Oliver and Boyd, 1928), p. 46.

4. [J. Naples], 'Manuscript Diary (The Diary of a Resurrectionist)', held at the Royal College of Surgeons of England, London; Evidence and Report of Select Committee on Anatomy, 1828.

5. Hurren, 'A Pauper Dead-House'; MacDonald, *Possessing the Dead*. See also Knox, 'The Body Politic', for an account of activities in Newcastle-upon-Tyne.

6. Richardson, *Death, Dissection and the Destitute*, pp. 104 and 311; MacDonald, *Possessing the Dead*, p. 22.

7. J. W. von Archenholz, *A Picture of England*, 2 vols (Dublin: P. Byrne, 1791), vol. 2, pp. 154–5.

8. J. Lane has noted that 'as a deterrent, many women found guilty of infanticide were sentenced to be anatomized after execution'; *The Making of the English Patient: A Guide to Sources for the Social History of Medicine* (Stroud: Sutton, 2000), p. 64. Of course total numbers were actually very small: of 200 women indicted for murder in Yorkshire, Northumberland, Cumberland and Westmorland between 1720 and 1800, only six were found guilty and only two were hanged; see M. Jackson, *New-Born Child Murder* (Manchester: Manchester University Press, 1996), p. 3.

9. W. Petty, *The Petty Papers* (New York: A. M. Kelley, 1967), pp. 157–67.

10. M. Davidson, *Medicine in Oxford: A Historical Romance* (Oxford: Basil Blackwell, 1953), p. 35. Hearne's point is supported by the archaeological evidence noted later.

11. K. Dewhurst, *Willis' Oxford Casebook* (Oxford: Sandford, 1981), p. 35.

12. Davidson, *Medicine in Oxford*, p. 157.

13. A. Clark (ed.), *The Life and Times of Anthony à Wood* (London: Oxford University Press, 1961), pp. 58–9.

14. C. Boardman, *Oxfordshire Sinners and Villains* (Oxford: Oxfordshire Record Office, 1994), pp. 118–19.

15. B. Bailey, *The Resurrection Men: A History of the Trade in Corpses* (London: Macdonald, 1991), p. 34.

16. Hearne, *Remarks and Collections*, vol. 7 (1906), p. 228.

17. Ibid., vol. 10 (1915), pp. 313–15.

18. T. R. Forbes, 'To be Dissected and Anatomized', *Journal of the History of Medicine and Allied Sciences*, 36 (1981), pp. 490–2, on p. 490.

19. Sinclair and Robb-Smith, *A Short History of Anatomical Teaching in Oxford*, p. 11.

20. *Jackson's Oxford Journal*, 4 May 1754.

21. *Jackson's Oxford Journal*, 28 March 1761.

22. J. R. Green and G. Roberson, *Studies in Oxford History Chiefly in the Eighteenth Century* (Oxford: Clarendon Press, 1901), p. 93.

23. Oxford Record Office (hereafter ORO), QSP 1/1, Calendar of Prisoners 1778–1844.

24. Dr Lee (1694–1755) graduated BM from Oxford in 1722; fellow of the Royal College of Physicians, 1732; appointed physician to Frederick, Prince of Wales, 1739.

25. Sinclair and Robb-Smith, *A Short History of Anatomical Teaching in Oxford*, p. 8.

26. Christ Church College, MS Estates, 127, nos. 216 and 218.

27. Christ Church College, Visitations of Dr Lee's Anatomy School.

28. A further source of legal dissection material was available to anatomists from those prisoners dying a 'natural' death on board the much-feared prison hulks between 1770 and 1857. One third of the hulk prisoners died and were 'buried in unconsecrated ground alongside the Thames, or sent for dissection, as a sideline which, according to one former prisoner, earned the hulk doctors five or six pounds a corpse'; J. A. Sharpe, *Judicial Punishment in England* (London: Faber, 1990), p. 53. This resource was of little use

to anatomists outside the metropolis until after the Anatomy Act was passed, when it became one of the few sources available to doctors in Oxford. This will therefore be examined in further detail in Chapter 4.

29. *Manchester Guardian*, 26 August 1826. In fact the physicians and surgeons of the infirmary were certainly expecting a body to be delivered to them on 23 August, which suggests there was a change of plan; see MRI, Minutes of Special Medical Committee 1822–47, 23 August 1826.

30. *Manchester Guardian*, 15 September 1827.

31. *Manchester Guardian*, 22 March 1828.

32. It would appear that the location of the assizes in Lancaster left the Manchester anatomists without a guaranteed source of bodies, even from the few available through the Murder Act.

33. *Manchester Guardian*, 19 March 1831.

34. Founder of Great Windmill School, 1746.

35. F. W. Jordan, *Life of J. Jordan, Surgeon: And an Account of the Rise and Progress of the Medical Schools in Manchester with Some Particulars of the Life of E. Stephens* (Manchester: Sherratt and Hughes, 1904), p. 55

36. F. C. Waite, 'A Century and a Quarter of Medical Education in Cleveland', unpublished manuscript, 1938, Cleveland Historical Sciences Library; quoted in Bonner, *Becoming a Physician*, p. 215.

37. 'Stealing Dead Bodies', in *Anecdotes of Eminent Persons Comprising Also Many Interesting Remains of Literature and Biography with Some Original Letters of Distinguished Characters*, 2 vols (London: Samuel Bagster, 1813), vol. 2, pp. 30–4, on p. 32.

38. Rosner, *Medical Education in the Age of Improvement*, p. 49.

39. Bell, *Letters on Professional Character and Manners*, p. 579.

40. Lawrence, 'Alexander Monro Primus', p. 201.

41. Ibid., p. 209.

42. Hearne, *Remarks and Collections*, vol. 8 (1907), p. 156. .

43. Ibid., vol. 5 (1901), p. 59.

44. ORO, PAR/207/2/A1/1, St Martin Carfax Vestry Minutes 1762–1843, 28 and 29 October 1798.

45. ORO, PAR/189/8/F2/1, All Saints Vestry Minutes, 27 April 1808.

46. Bellers, *An Essay Towards the Improvement of Physick in Twelve Proposals*, p. 14.

47. Quarrell and Quarrell, *Oxford in 1710 from the Travels of Zacharias Conrad von Uffenbach*, p. 24.

48. Hearne, *Remarks and Collections*, vol. 2 (1886), p. 203.

49. Ibid., p. 382.

50. Ibid., vol. 8 (1907), pp. 156–7.

51. J. A. Bennett, S. A. Johnston and A. V. Simcock, *Solomon's House in Oxford: New Finds from the First Museum* (Oxford: Museum of the History of Science, 2000), p. 26.

52. Ibid., p. 55.

53. Ibid., pp. 50–1, and personal communication.

54. I am very grateful to Mark Steadman, curator of the 'Solomon's House' exhibition at the Museum for the History of Science, Oxford, for sharing his thoughts on these matters.

55. R. T. Gunther, *Early Science in Oxford*, 3 vols (Oxford: Oxford University Press, 1925), vol. 3, p. 117.

56. ORO, QSP 1/2, Calendar of Prisoners 1822–40.

57. *Jackson's Oxford Journal*, 16 October 1830.

58. *Jackson's Oxford Journal*, 19 November 1831.
59. E. Tatham, 'A New Address to the Free and Independent Members of Convocation', quoted in Robb-Smith, 'Medical Education', p. 567.
60. Select Committee on Medical Education, 1834, Q4537.
61. *Manchester Guardian*, 20 December 1823.
62. G. A. G. Mitchell, 'Resurrection Days', *Manchester University Gazette*, 27 (1848), pp. 150–4, on p. 152.
63. J. Jordan, 'A Case of Obliteration of the Aorta', *North of England Medical and Surgical Journal*, 1 (1830), pp. 101–4, on p. 104.
64. E. Stephens, 'Notes', in Jordan, *Life of J. Jordan, Surgeon*, pp. 127–35.
65. *Memoir of Thomas Turner*, p. 88.
66. T. Turner, *On Poisons and Suspended Animation* (Manchester, 1823); T. Turner, *Outlines of a Course of Lectures on the Laws of Animal Life and the Application of Anatomy, Physiology and Other Sciences to the Principles and Practice of Medicine and Surgery* (Manchester, 1825); *A Practical Treatise on the Arterial System*; T. Turner, *Anatomico-Chirurgical Observations on Dislocation of the Astragulus* (Worcester, 1843).
67. T. Fawdington, *A Catalogue Descriptive Chiefly of the Morbid Preparations Contained in the Museum of the Manchester Theatre of Anatomy and Medicine, Marsden Street, with Occasional Explanatory Remarks* (Manchester: Harrison and Crossfield, 1833).
68. Ibid., pp. 41 and 44.
69. Ibid., p. 26.
70. W. Brockbank, *The Honorary Medical Staff of the Manchester Royal Infirmary 1830–1948* (Manchester: Manchester University Press, 1965), p. 11.
71. MUJRL, MMC, Items 24 and 40, catalogue of the preparations in the Museum of the Mount Street School belonging to Joseph Jordan.
72. MUJRL, MMC, Item 63.
73. This lends support to the possibility that post-mortems could be more extensive than relatives realized, which is discussed in this chapter.
74. *Manchester Guardian*, 1 January 1825.
75. *The Trial of John Eaton* (Manchester: J. Pratt, 1827).
76. *Voice of the People*, 29 January 1831.
77. See, for example, *Manchester Guardian*, 3 January 1824; 29 October 1824; 4 March 1826; 2 August 1828; 6 February 1830; 27 February 1830. Much of the press coverage relates only to incidents of discovery, and so bodysnatching activity in Manchester is likely to have been substantially greater than this evidence suggests.
78. *Manchester Guardian*, 21 February 1824.
79. *Manchester Guardian*, 29 July 1826.
80. *Lancaster Gazette*, 7 October 1826.
81. *Manchester Guardian*, 29 October 1825.
82. Richardson, *Death, Dissection and the Destitute*, p. 135.
83. Mitchell, 'Resurrection Days', p. 150.
84. *Manchester Guardian*, 23 January 1830.
85. *Voice of the People*, 29 January 1831.
86. *Manchester Guardian*, 6 February 1830.
87. *Poor Man's Advocate*, 31 March 1832 (the resulting libel case was covered on 8 September 1832; Doherty was sentenced to one month's imprisonment).
88. *Poor Man's Advocate*, 9 June 1832.

89. J. Reinarz, 'The Age of Museum Medicine: The Rise and Fall of the Medical Museum at Birmingham's School of Medicine', *Social History of Medicine*, 18 (2005), pp. 419–37, on p. 422.
90. H. Alford, 'The Bristol Infirmary in my Student Days 1822–28', *Bristol Medico-Chirurgical Journal*, 8 (1890), pp. 165–91, on p. 167.
91. M. Fido, *Body-Snatchers: A History of the Resurrectionists, 1742–1832* (London: Weidenfeld and Nicolson, 1988), p. 40.
92. MacDonald, *Possessing the Dead*, p. 22.
93. Maulitz, *Morbid Appearances*, pp. 138–9.
94. See V. McMahon, 'Reading the Body: Dissection and the "Murder" of Sarah Stout, Hertfordshire, 1699', *Social History of Medicine*, 19 (2006), pp. 19–35, for an interesting discussion.
95. Farre, *An Apology for British Anatomy*, p. 8.
96. I. A. Burney, *Bodies of Evidence: Medicine and the Politics of the English Inquest, 1830–1926* (Baltimore, MD and London: Johns Hopkins University Press, 2000), pp. 55 and 193.
97. Mann, *Recollections of my Early and Professional Life*, p. 106.
98. Ibid., p. 107.
99. MacDonald, *Possessing the Dead*, pp. 96–104.
100. Today the numbers of hospital post-mortems are at an all time low, and pathologists use the coronial autopsy to teach pathology to junior doctors. See 'Drop in Hospital Autopsies Restricts Hands-on Learning', *BMA News*, 1 December 2001; K. Mattick, R. Marshall and J. Bligh, 'Tissue Pathology in Undergraduate Medical Education: Atrophy or Evolution?', *Journal of Pathology*, 203 (2004), pp. 871–6; G. O'Grady 'Death of the Teaching Autopsy', *British Medical Journal*, 327 (2003), pp. 802–4; 'Cadavers Down to a Skeletal Supply', *BMA News*, 21 April 2007, p. 8.
101. Richardson, *Death, Dissection and the Destitute*, p. 44.
102. Ibid., pp. 104 and 311.
103. H. Marland, *Medicine and Society in Wakefield and Huddersfield 1780–1870* (Cambridge: Cambridge University Press 1987), p. 127.
104. Ibid., p. 156.
105. G. B. Risse, *Hospital Life in Enlightenment Scotland* (Cambridge: Cambridge University Press, 1986), p. 263.
106. Lawrence, *Charitable Knowledge*, p. 124.
107. Radcliffe Infirmary, RI C/I/1, Board of Governors Minutes, 7 February 1780.
108. Radcliffe Infirmary, RI C/I/5, 9 October 1816.
109. Radcliffe Infirmary, RI C/1/1, 22 October 1795.
110. Radcliffe Infirmary, RI C/I/5, 18 October 1821.
111. Radcliffe Infirmary, RI C/I/7, 3 May 1837, numbers of burials:

1830	1
1831	7
1832	10
1833	10
1834	12
1835	3
1836	2

112. Radcliffe Infirmary, RI C/I/1, 7 March 1775.

113. MRI, Minutes of Manchester Infirmary 1818, p. 153; and Manchester Medical Collection, biographical files, MMC/2/Fawdington.

114. T. Fawdington, *A Case of Melanosis, with General Observations on the Pathology of this Interesting Disease* (London: Longman; Manchester: Robinson, 1826), p. 49.

115. W. Brockbank, *Portrait of a Hospital* (London: William Heinemann, 1952), p. 57.

116. Forbes, 'To be Dissected and Anatomized', p. 492.

117. *Lancet*, 2 (1828), p. 153.

118. *Jackson's Oxford Journal*, 7 February 1829.

119. J. McManners, *Death and the Enlightenment: Changing Attitudes to Death among Christians and Unbelievers in Eighteenth-Century France* (Oxford: Oxford University Press, 1981), p. 145.

120. Richardson, *Death, Dissection and the Destitute*, p. 99.

121. *Poor Man's Advocate*, 31 March 1832.

122. Richardson, *Death, Dissection and the Destitute*, p. 14.

123. G. A. Walker, *Gatherings from Grave Yards: Particularly Those of London; with a Concise History of the Modes of Interment among Different Nations from the Earliest Period. And a Detail of Dangerous and Fatal Results Produced by the Unwise and Revolting Custom of Inhuming the Dead in the Midst of the Living* (London: Longman, 1839), p. 188.

124. *Times*, 17 February 1824. Interestingly, Dr Nathan Alcock (1707–79), Oxford University praelector in anatomy and anatomy lecturer at Jesus College, 'lieth interred in a leaden coffin'; J. Smith, *Some Memoirs of the Life of Dr Nathan Alcock* (London: Buckland and Co., 1780), p. 61.

125. MUJRL, MMC/14/10.

126. J. S. Curl, *The Victorian Celebration of Death* (Newton Abbott: David and Charles, 1972), p. 60.

127. J. Rugg, 'A New Burial Form and its Meanings: Cemetery Establishment in the First Half of the Nineteenth Century', in M. Cox (ed.), *Grave Concerns: Death and Burial in England 1700–1850* (York: Council for British Archaeology, 1998), pp. 44–53, on p. 46.

128. Ibid., p. 46.

129. *Manchester Guardian*, 21 February 1824.

130. Engels, *The Condition of the Working Class in England*, p. 315.

131. National Archives, Home Office Records (hereafter NA, HO) 44/1, 5 February 1820.

132. *Trial of John Eaton*, p. 3.

133. Ibid., pp. 7–8.

134. Ibid., p. 8.

135. T. Rowlandson, *The Persevering Surgeon*, painting, late eighteenth century. For an interesting discussion of art and anatomy, see F. Haslam, *From Hogarth to Rowlandson: Medicine in Art in Eighteenth-Century Britain* (Liverpool: Liverpool University Press, 1996); and Porter, *Bodies Politic*.

136. *Times*, 9 December 1822.

137. E. Ravenscroft, *The Anatomist; or Sham Doctor* (London: John Cawthorn, 1807).

138. Recent anatomy/pathology scandals have come to light when families became aware of the reality of post-mortem examination, including the removal of whole organs due to confusion over the terms 'tissue' and 'specimen'.

139. *Times*, 5 October 1839, p. 6.

140. *Lancet*, 1 (2 November 1839), p. 206.

141. *Jackson's Oxford Journal*, 27 November 1830.

142. Archer, *Social Unrest and Popular Protest in England*, p. 20.

143. *Oxford University and City Herald*, 11 September 1830.
144. *Oxford University and City Herald*, 25 September 1830.
145. ORO, CPZ/15, Otmoor Enclosure Papers.
146. Ibid.
147. National Archives, Otmoor Enclosure Papers, TS 11/1031/4433.
148. Bodleian Library, MS Dep. b. 48, Oxon Lent Assizes 1832, Brief for the Prosecution, p. 6.
149. Lawrence, 'Anatomy and Address', p. 212.

3 The Anatomy Act and the Poor

1. Evidence for this can be gleaned from a variety of medical journals, including the *Lancet*, and local and national papers. I have surveyed the *London Medical Gazette* in detail from 1827 to 1832. Particular examples include: 8 December 1827; 16 February 1828; 13 September 1828; 24 January 1829; 21 March 1829; 6 June 1829; 13 June 1829; 8 August 1829; 27 February 1830; 13 March 1830; 10 December 1831; 4 February 1832; 25 February 1832.
2. Richardson, *Death, Dissection and the Destitute*, p. 107.
3. Jordan, *Life of J. Jordan, Surgeon*, p. 55.
4. SCA, appendix no. 23.
5. SCA, Qs 1374–9, pp. 116–17.
6. SCA, Q 1392, p. 117.
7. SCA, Q 27, p. 155.
8. SCA, Q 1, p. 14.
9. SCA, Q 980, p. 85.
10. SCA, Q 219, p. 33.
11. SCA, Q 171, p. 28.
12. SCA, Qs 261–2, p. 36.
13. SCA, Evidence of Astley Cooper, Q 53, p. 19.
14. SCA, Qs 997–8, p. 87.
15. SCA, Evidence Q 40.
16. SCA, Evidence Q 50.
17. SCA, Q 58, p. 19; *London Medical Gazette*, 2 (13 September 1828), p. 472.
18. SCA, Q 143, p. 26.
19. SCA, Q 142, p. 26.
20. SCA, Q 192, p. 31.
21. SCA, Q 287, p. 37.
22. Member of the Royal College of Surgeons, 1822; ran Webb Street Anatomy School from 1822 until its closure in 1830s, which was caused by lack of bodies under the Anatomy Act; appointed lecturer in anatomy and physiology at St Thomas's; dissected Richard Carlisle on philosopher's own request, 1843; fellow of the Royal College of Surgeons, 1843.
23. SCA, Q 397, p. 45.
24. SCA, appendix no. 8.
25. Richardson, *Death, Dissection and the Destitute*, p. 121.
26. SCA, Evidence of Sir Astley Cooper, Q 67, p. 19.
27. Guthrie, *A Letter ... on Anatomy*, p. 16.
28. SCA, Q 146, p. 26.

29. SCA, Q 149, p. 26.
30. SCA, Qs 197–8, p. 31.
31. Guthrie, *A Letter ... on Anatomy*, p. 9.
32. SCA, appendix no. 8.
33. SCA, p. 12.
34. At the end of 1828 the activities of William Burke (1792–1829) and William Hare (1792/1804–62) in Edinburgh were discovered. They had murdered poor vagrants from November 1827, selling sixteen bodies to the anatomist Robert Knox (1791–1862). Burke was hanged and his body dissected, while Hare was pardoned for giving evidence against his accomplice. Despite the anger of the Edinburgh poor, no charges were brought against Knox, although the murderers claimed that he was present when several bodies were delivered and had commented on their freshness; Richardson, *Death, Dissection and the Destitute*, pp. 131–43.
35. *London Medical Gazette*, 4 (6 June 1829), p. 24.
36. *Lancet*, 2 (1828–9), p. 241.
37. *Lancet*, 1 (1828–9), p. 756.
38. *Lancet*, 2 (16 March 1829), p. 15. In fact, this was to prove a disappointing source for Oxford and Cambridge universities. This will be discussed in the following chapter.
39. *London Medical Gazette*, 5 (27 February 1830), p. 698.
40. Ibid.
41. The story is covered extensively in S. Wise, *The Italian Boy: Murder and Grave-Robbery in 1830s London* (London: Jonathan Cape, 2004).
42. *Voice of the People*, 9 April 1831.
43. *Voice of the People*, 19 February 1831.
44. Hansard's Parliamentary Debates, 2nd ser., 9, 17 January 1832.
45. Hansard, 24 January 1832, p. 826.
46. Ibid., p. 828.
47. Hansard, 11 May 1832, p. 896.
48. Hansard, 17 January 1832, p. 579.
49. Ibid., p. 578.
50. Hansard, 27 February 1832, pp. 832–4.
51. *Jackson's Oxford Journal*, 12 February 1831; and Hansard, 2 February 1832, p. 1185.
52. Hansard, 3rd ser., 10, 15 February 1832, pp. 377–8.
53. 2 & 3 Gul. IV c. 75: An Act for Regulating Schools of Anatomy, 1832, clause 7.
54. In fact the dissection of murderers must have continued when bodies from the prison hulks were utilized, notably by Oxford and Cambridge universities; see Chapter 4.
55. Richardson, *Death, Dissection and the Destitute*, pp. 219–22.
56. Guthrie, *A Letter ... on Anatomy*, p. 26.
57. *Poor Man's Advocate*, 15 September 1832.
58. Durey, *The Return of the Plague*, p. 168.
59. R. J. Morris, *Cholera 1832: The Social History of an Epidemic* (London: Croom Helm, 1976), pp. 43–4.
60. Radcliffe Infirmary, RI, 1832 Cholera File.
61. Richardson, *Death, Dissection and the Destitute*, p. 360 n. 45.
62. Sinclair and Robb-Smith, *A Short History of Anatomical Teaching in Oxford*, p. 45.
63. Bodleian Library, MSS.Top.Oxon.d.245, Oxford Board of Health, p. 265.
64. Bodleian Library, MSS.Top.Oxon.c.272, Oxford Board of Health.

65. V. Thomas, *Memorials of the Malignant Cholera in Oxford 1832* (Oxford: W. Baxter, 1835), p. 22.
66. Radcliffe Infirmary, RI, 1832 Cholera File, Oxford Board of Health, 2 August 1832.
67. Bodleian Library, MSS.Top.Oxon.c.272, Oxford Board of Health, p. 199.
68. Manchester Central Reference Library (hereafter MCRL), M9/36/1–2, Manchester Board of Health Papers 1831–3, 28 June 1832.
69. Ibid., 17 August 1832.
70. H. Gaulter, *The Origins and Progress of the Malignant Cholera in Manchester* (London: Longman and Co., 1833), p. 35.
71. Ibid., pp. 38–9.
72. Ibid., p. 137.
73. *Manchester Guardian*, 8 September 1832.
74. *Jackson's Oxford Journal*, 8 September 1832.
75. *Poor Man's Advocate* 15 September 1832.
76. *Poor Man's Advocate*, 14 July 1832.
77. NA, PC1/93, Central Board of Health letter book, 22 November 1831.
78. S. Gaskell, 'Cholera in Manchester', *Edinburgh Medical and Surgical Journal*, 40 (1833), pp. 52–65, on p. 56.
79. Burrell and Gill, 'The Liverpool Cholera Epidemic of 1832'.
80. E. C. Midwinter, *Social Administration in Lancashire 1830–1860* (Manchester: Manchester University Press, 1969), p. 71.
81. Burrell and Gill, 'The Liverpool Cholera Epidemic of 1832', p. 485.
82. *Liverpool Chronicle*, 2 June 1832.
83. Burrell and Gill, 'The Liverpool Cholera Epidemic on 1832', p. 494.
84. Durey, *The Return of the Plague*, pp. 158–9.
85. National Archives, Anatomy Office Out-Letter Books (hereafter NA, MH) 74/12, 1832–5, letter to Thomas Turner in Manchester, 16 March 1833.
86. *Jackson's Oxford Journal*, 7 December 1833.
87. NA, MH 74/12, 4 December 1833.
88. hereafter NA, HO 83/1, 9 December 1833.
89. *The Christian's Appeal against the Poor Law Amendment Act* (broadsheet), 1834, quoted in Richardson, *Death, Dissection and the Destitute*, pp. 264–5.
90. Donnelly, 'The Destruction of the Sheffield School of Anatomy in 1835', p. 171.
91. Ibid., p. 170; S. Roberts, *The Lecturers Lectured, and the Dissectors Dissected* (Sheffield, 1834), p. 3.
92. NA, MH 74/10, 1842–79, letter of 7 May 1847.
93. Ibid., letter of 24 May 1847.
94. D. Thompson, *The Early Chartists* (London: Macmillan, 1971), p. xi.
95. A. Crossley, 'A History of the County of Oxford', in C. R. Elrington (ed.), *The Victoria History of the Counties of England*, vol. 4 (Oxford: Oxford University Press, 1979), pp. 74–180, on p. 81.
96. M. Graham, *Images of Victorian Oxford* (Stroud: Alan Sutton, 1992), p. 105.

4 The Working of the Anatomy Act in Oxford and Manchester

1. Inspector of anatomy for England and Wales, 1832–42; and inspector for Scotland, 1836–42.
2. NA, MH 74/10, 11 January 1834.

3. NA, MH 74/12, 1 October 1833; regrettably the register does not appear to have survived.
4. NA, MH 74/12, 5 November 1832 and 28 September 1832.
5. This campaign is covered extensively in Richardson, *Death, Dissection and the Destitute*, pp. 246–9.
6. NA, MH 74/36, 30 January 1882.
7. NA, HO 45 9341–22233/1.
8. *Lancet*, 1 (11 December 1841), pp. 377–81, on p. 380.
9. E. R. Lankester, *Second Annual Report of the Central District of Middlesex* (London, 1865), p. 196.
10. Richardson, *Death, Dissection and the Destitute*, p. 242.
11. Great Windmill Street, Little Windmill Street, Webb Street, Dean Street, Little Dean Street, Chapel Street, Howland Street, Aldersgate Street.
12. Guy's, London, St Bartholomew's, St Thomas's.
13. Charing Cross, King's, Middlesex, St George's, St Mary's, University College and Westminster; see Richardson, *Death, Dissection and the Destitute*, appendix 1; and NA, MH 74/16, 19 July 1871.
14. NA, MH 74/12, 15 January 1835.
15. Richardson, *Death, Dissection and the Destitute*, p. 245.
16. LSA; member of the Royal College of Surgeons; honorary surgeon at Manchester Royal Infirmary, 1837–43.
17. Fellow of the Royal College of Surgeons; surgeon to Salford and Pendleton Royal Dispensary.
18. K. A. Webb, 'The Development of the Medical Profession in Manchester 1750–1860' (PhD thesis, University of Manchester, 1988).
19. Fellow of the Royal College of Surgeons; honorary surgeon at Manchester Royal Infirmary, 1847–71.
20. Fellow of the Royal College of Surgeons; honorary surgeon at Manchester Royal Infirmary, 1847–76; professor at Owens College.
21. Richardson, *Death, Dissection and the Destitute*, p. 241.
22. NA, MH 74/12.
23. See Appendix, Table I.
24. NA, MH 74/12, 12 September 1832.
25. *Manchester Guardian*, 27 October 1832.
26. NA, MH 74/12, 16 March 1833.
27. NA, MH 74/12, 22 April 1833.
28. NA, MH 74/13, 13 November 1838.
29. NA, MH 74/12, 12 September 1832.
30. Jordan, *Life of J. Jordan, Surgeon*, pp. 52 and 83.
31. Ibid., p. 44.
32. Ibid., p. 83.
33. NA, MH 74/10, 4 October 1855. See Appendix, Table I: it seems that bodies continued to be allocated to Bridge Street, Jordan's home.
34. *Manchester Guardian* clipping from 1840; in MUJRL, MMC, Thomas Turner file.
35. NA, MH 74/10, 12 January 1849.
36. *Memoir of Thomas Turner*, p. 155.
37. NA, MH 74/10, 1 November 1850.
38. Ibid., 21 November 1851.

39. Ibid., 4 December 1851.
40. Provincial Inspector of Anatomy, 1844.
41. It seems likely that this individual is William Roberts. His early campaign against the Anatomy Inspector, Somerville, is well documented in Richardson, *Death, Dissection and the Destitute*, pp. 246–50.
42. NA, MH 74/10, 7 May 1847.
43. Ibid., 18 and 20 November 1851.
44. Ibid., 22 December 1851.
45. See Appendix, Tables II and III for cadaver and student numbers where known.
46. NA, MH 74/10, 26 January 1852.
47. Ibid., 16 February 1852.
48. Probably William Smith (1817–75), LSA, member of the Royal College of Surgeons; nephew of Thomas Turner; surgeon at the Manchester Royal Infirmary, 1847–75; professor of anatomy and physiology at Owens College, 1873.
49. NA, MH 74/10, 1 and 4 September 1852.
50. Ibid., 25 October 1852.
51. Ibid., 22 December 1852.
52. Ibid., 23 December 1852.
53. Ibid., 19 November 1856.
54. Ibid., January 1857.
55. Ibid., 13 February 1857.
56. Ibid., 21 December 1857.
57. Ibid., 28 October 1858.
58. Ibid., 4 November 1858.
59. Ibid., 24 November 1858.
60. Ibid., 29 November 1858.
61. Ibid., 20 November, 1863.
62. See Appendix, Table I.
63. NA, MH 74/10, 14 December 1863.
64. Ibid., October and November 1864.
65. Ibid., 22 May 1866.
66. Minutes of Council, School of Medicine, Leeds University Archive; quoted in Bonner, *Becoming a Physician*, p. 225.
67. S. T. Anning and K. J. Walls, *A History of the Leeds School of Medicine: One and a Half Centuries 1831–1981* (Leeds: Leeds University Press, 1982), pp. 21–2.
68. Ibid., p. 57.
69. MCRL, M10/808, Hulme Letters, 1 August 1834. I am very grateful to Steve King for sharing his research on the Hulme letters.
70. MCRL, M327/1/2/13, Withington Workhouse Register of Burials.
71. MCRL, M327/2/5/1, Withington Workhouse Register of Burials.
72. *Lancet*, 1 (19 June 1909), p. 1786.
73. See Appendix, Table II.
74. Hurren, 'A Pauper Dead-House'.
75. MD University College, 1859; praelector in physiology at Cambridge, 1870; first professor of physiology at Cambridge, 1883–1903; knighted 1899; MP for University of London, 1900.

76. London MB, 1840; MRCS, 1841; LSA, 1842; surgeon at Addenbrooke's, 1842; fellow of the Royal College of Surgeons, 1844; deputy to professor of anatomy at Cambridge, 1847; professor of human anatomy, 1866–83; knighted 1891.

77. Lee's Reader in Anatomy at Oxford, 1857; Linacre Professor of Anatomy and Physiology, 1860–81.

78. MD, 1851; Waynflete Professor of Physiology at Oxford, 1882; Regius Professor of Medicine at Oxford, 1895–1904; baronet 1899.

79. Educated at Edinburgh University, MB MRCS 1880; demonstrator of anatomy to William Turner at Edinburgh University.

80. NA, MH 74/13, letter to John Hopps, York, 13 October 1835.

81. NA, HO 83/1, 3 October 1833.

82. Ibid., 18 March 1835.

83. NA, MH 74/13, 28 January 1836.

84. Ibid., 15 March 1836; NA, HO 83/1, 23 October 1835. (Oxford and Cambridge universities sent their concerns directly to the Home Secretary or Chancellor of the Exchequer.)

85. NA, MH 74/14, 13 December 1841.

86. Weatherall, *Gentlemen, Scientists and Doctors*, p. 45.

87. NA, MH 74/15, 30 November 1842. At the 1828 Select Committee on Anatomy, David Arnott, surgeon on the *Grampus*, stated his enthusiasm for conducting post-mortems on board the hulk and his hope that this would continue after legislation; SCA 1828, Qs 854–64.

88. NA, MH 74/15, AnReport of the Metropolitan Inspector, 31 December 1842.

89. NA, MH 74/12, letter of 5 September 1833 to John Fieldsen in Oxford, and letter of 16 February 1833 to R. T. Hunt in Manchester are two relevant examples among many others in the National Archives.

90. *Lancet*, 2 (21 April 1829), p. 175.

91. See Appendix, Table I.

92. William Clark, Cambridge professor of anatomy, 1817–66.

93. NA, MH 74/13, 9 November 1836.

94. NA, MH 74/14, 10 November 1841.

95. Ibid., 1 December 1841.

96. Ibid., 6 December 1841.

97. NA, MH 74/15, letter to A Waddington, Home Office, dated January 1853.

98. NA, MH 74/15, 23 January 1844.

99. NA, MH 74/10, 28 September 1852.

100. Ibid., 18 October 1853.

101. Ibid., 6 December 1855 and 9 April 1860.

102. Ibid., 15 April 1861.

103. Ibid., 8 October 1863.

104. See Appendix, Table II.

105. Christ Church College, MS Estates 127, 24 December 1836.

106. RI/C/1/9, 22 January 1840.

107. Ibid., 11 December 1839.

108. NA, MH 74/10, 10 August 1861.

109. Ibid., 5 December 1864. The returns of bodies received by schools of anatomy in the Anatomy Inspectorate records note that only one body was received by Oxford; see Appendix, Table I.

110. NA, MH 74/10, 13 January 1865.
111. Ibid., 28 October 1872.
112. NA, MH 74/11, 23 October 1879.
113. NA, MH 74/10, 30 October 1872, 8 March 1873 and 25 September 1876; the returns from anatomy schools to the Anatomy Inspectorate.
114. RI/C/1/18, 29 December 1886.
115. RI/C/1/20, July–August 1899.
116. For example, see the cases of Mrs Hale and the Thames Board of Guardians, 1898, and of Dora Atkins, 1899, both in RI/C/1/20.
117. RI/C/1/20, 3 August 1898.
118. RI/C/1/21, 4 October 1899.
119. ORO, AU/PLU/A1/003, Headington Board of Guardians Minute Book, 7 November 1861.
120. NA, MH 74/11, 23 October 1879.
121. See Appendix, Table I.
122. NA, MH 74/11, 15 October 1896.
123. Ibid.
124. Oxford University Archives, Human Anatomy file (hereafter OUA, HA89).
125. C. Keetley and R. Wharry, *The Student's and Junior Practitioner's Guide to the Medical Profession*, 2nd edn (London: Balliere, Tindall and Cox, 1885), p. 50.
126. OUA, HA89.
127. NA, MH 74/38, 31 July 1905.
128. OUA, HA89.
129. OUA, HA89.
130. 'The Oxford Medical School', *British Medical Journal* (23 June 1906), pp. 1–15, on p. 10.
131. Oxford City Archives (hereafter OCA), C/ENG/1/A7/1, Rose Hill Cemetery Register of Burials; OCA, C/ENG/1/A10/2, Wolvercote Cemetery Register of Burials; OCA, C/ENG/1/A1/2, Botley Cemetery Register of Burials.
132. Hurren, 'A Pauper Dead-House', p. 91. Whitechapel supplied one body interred at Rose Hill. See Appendix, Table III for complete figures.
133. *Hospital*, 12 February 1910, p. 579.
134. OCA, Reports of English Cemeteries and of the Oxford Sub-Committee, Letters etc., c.2.29, Minutes (1889–1915), 11 February 1915.
135. OUA, HA89.
136. Weatherall, *Gentlemen, Scientists and Doctors*, p. 56.

5 Medical Education in Oxford and Manchester after the Anatomy Act

1.   M. Baillie, *Morbid Anatomy* (1793), quoted in Bonner, *Becoming a Physician*, p. 147.
2.   R. Dunglison, *The Medical Student: Or Aids to the Study of Medicine* (Philadelphia, PA: Carey, Lea and Blanchard, 1837), quoted in Bonner, *Becoming a Physician*, pp. 157–8.
3.   G. L. Geison, 'Social and Institutional Factors in the Stagnancy of English Physiology, 1840–1870', *Bulletin of the History of Medicine*, 46 (1972), pp. 30–58, on p. 30.
4.   M. Foster, *On Medical Education at Cambridge* (London: Macmillan, 1878), p. 16.
5.   *British Medical Journal*, 1 (1883), p. 1188.
6.   Geison, 'Social and Institutional Factors', p. 35.

7. Atlay, *Sir Henry Wentworth Acland*, p. 169.
8. H. W. Acland, 'Remarks on the Extension of Education at the University of Oxford, in a Letter to the Rev. W. Jacobson, Regius Professor of Divinity and Canon of Christ Church Oxford', in Atlay, *Sir Henry Wentworth Acland,* p. 248.
9. Ibid., p. 334.
10. Bodleian Library, MS Acland d.62, 3 February 1852.
11. Reinarz, 'The Age of Museum Medicine', p. 424.
12. Sinclair and Robb-Smith, *A Short History of Anatomical Teaching in Oxford*, p. 63.
13. P. K. Underhill, 'Science, Professionalism and the Development of Medical Education in England: An Historical Sociology' (PhD thesis, University of Edinburgh, 1987), p. 172.
14. *British Medical Journal* (5 January 1878); and (12 January 1878).
15. Chair of zoology at University College London, 1875; Linacre Chair of Comparative Anatomy at Oxford University, 1891; director of natural history at the British Museum, 1898; KCB 1907.
16. Robb-Smith, 'Medical Education', p. 577.
17. *British Medical Journal* (16 February 1878), p. 244.
18. T. M. Romano, *Making Medicine Scientific: John Burdon-Sanderson and the Culture of Victorian Science* (Baltimore, MD: Johns Hopkins University, 2002), p. 140.
19. *British Medical Journal* (2 February 1878), p. 160.
20. E. R. Lankester, 'An Address to the Medical Department of University College on Opening Session 1878–9', *British Medical Journal* (1878), pp. 501–7, on p. 506.
21. Oxford University Archives, Hebdomadal Council Papers (hereafter OUA, HC/1/5), memorandum no. 4, November 1874.
22. 'Oxford and Cambridge: A Contrast', *British Medical Journal*, 1 (1879) p. 197.
23. J. S. Sharkey, *The University of Oxford and Medical Education* (n.p., 1879), p. 3.
24. OUA, HC/1/5, letter to Vice-Chancellor Liddell, 7 May 1873.
25. OUA, HC/1/5, note to Hebdomadal Council, 12 February 1879.
26. OUA, HC/1/5, Evidence to Committee on Medicine and Engineering, 1879.
27. Ibid.
28. St Bartholomew's consultant, 1871; president of the Royal College of Surgeons, 1875; vice-chancellor at the University of London, 1884–95.
29. A. J. Engel, *From Clergyman to Don: the Rise of the Academic Profession in Nineteenth-Century Oxford* (Oxford: Clarendon Press, 1983), p. 220.
30. OUA, HC/1/5.
31. Assistant physician to City of London Hospital; medical tutor at St Bartholomew's.
32. OUA, HC/1/5, 'The Proposed Establishment of a Medical School in Oxford', 29 April 1879.
33. Robb-Smith, 'Medical Education', p. 578.
34. Regius Professor of Greek at Oxford, 1855; master of Balliol College, 1870; vice-chancellor at Oxford University, 1882–6.
35. V. Quinn and J. Prest (eds), *Dear Miss Nightingale: A Selection of Benjamin Jowett's Letters to Florence Nightingale 1860–1893* (Oxford: Clarendon Press, 1987), p. 297.
36. Acland, *Oxford and Modern Medicine*, p. 10.
37. Dean of Christ Church, 1855–91.
38. Bodleian Library, MS Acland d.92, fols 49–54, B. Carpenter to Acland, 5 May 1885.
39. T. M. Romano, 'Gentlemanly versus Scientific Ideals: John Burdon-Sanderson, Medical Education and the Failure of the Oxford School of Physiology', *Bulletin of the History of Medicine*, 71 (1997), pp. 224–48, on p. 235.

40. Ibid., p. 240.
41. J. S. Burdon-Sanderson, *The School of Medical Science in Oxford* (Oxford: Horace Hart, 1892), p. 6.
42. Bodleian Library, MS Acland d.69, 1 June 1891, Letters from Dean Liddell. Henry Liddell was a close friend and supporter of Henry Acland.
43. Quinn and Prest (eds), *Dear Miss Nightingale*, p. 173.
44. From 1891.
45. Romano, *Making Medicine Scientific*, p. 363.
46. Bodleian Library, MS Acland d.69, 20 March 1892.
47. Romano, *Making Medicine Scientific*, p. 365.
48. W. D. Hemming, *The Medical Student's Guide* (London: Bailliere, Tindall and Cox, 1876), p. 2.
49. Anning, 'Provincial Medical Schools in the Nineteenth Century', p. 131.
50. Professor of natural history, anatomy and physiology, 1851; professor of natural history, 1872; professor of botany, 1880; emeritus professor 1892.
51. Bonner, *Becoming a Physician*, p. 247.
52. Honorary physician at Addenbrooke's, 1839–84; Regius Professor of Physic at Cambridge University, 1872–92; President of the General Medical Council, 1869–74; fellow of Royal College of Physicians, 1873; knighted 1887.
53. Weatherall, *Gentlemen, Scientists and Doctors*, p. 129.
54. Royal Commission Appointed to Inquire into the Medical Acts, 1882 (Cd 3259-1), p. xiii.
55. J. E. Morgan, *The Victoria University: Why are There No Medical Degrees?* (Manchester: J. E. Cornish, 1881), pp. 7–8.
56. Ibid., p. 9.
57. Ibid., p. 17.
58. Ibid., p. 19.
59. Hemming, *The Medical Student's Guide*, p. 7.
60. [Anon.], *The Victoria University of Manchester Medical School* (Manchester: Manchester University Press, 1908), p. 16.
61. Keetley and Wharry, *The Student's and Junior Practitioner's Guide*, p. 66.
62. C. Keetley, *The Student's Guide to the Medical Profession* (London: Macmillan, 1878), p. 20.
63. Oxford University Archives, 'Remarks by Dr Acland on a Draft Report to Committee of Hebdomadal Council on Engineering and Medicine', 5 November 1879.
64. A. H. T. Robb-Smith, *A Short History of the Radcliffe Infirmary* (Oxford: Church Army Press for the United Oxford Hospitals, 1970), p. 61.
65. RI/C/1/9, 8 January 1840.
66. Robb-Smith, 'Medical Education', p. 571.
67. Hemming, *The Medical Student's Guide*, p. 1.
68. *British Medical Journal* (26 January 1878), p. 141.
69. RI/C/1/10, 17 March 1846, p. 61.
70. Weatherall, *Gentlemen, Scientists and Doctors*, pp. 126–7.
71. *British Medical Journal*, 1 (1883), pp. 1188–9.
72. Acland, *Oxford and Modern Medicine*, p. 25.
73. Morgan, *The Victoria University*, pp. 17–19.
74. Foster, *On Medical Education at Cambridge*, p. 3.

75. Post-mortem rates at the Radcliffe Infirmary are presented in Appendix Table IV, but these have been poorly compiled and need to be treated with care.
76. For example, Birmingham Queens Medical School amalgamated with Mason College in 1892, and Bristol Medical School became a College Faculty in 1893.

6 Some Contemporary Parallels

1. *Mail Online*, 4 January 2011, at http://www.dailymail.co.uk/news/article-1343910/Gunther-von-Hagens-Dr-Death-plans-human-corpse-exhibition-grim-farewell.html [accessed 28 April 2013].
2. 'Alexander Sizonenko', at http://www.thetallestman.com/alexandersizonenko.htm [accessed 28 April 2013].
3. Moore, *The Knife Man*, p. 349.
4. *Guardian*, 23 January 2004, at www.guardian.co.uk/world/2004/jan/23/arts.china [accessed 28 April 2013]. The findings by *Der Spiegel* were also widely reported by the BBC and the *Telegraph* at the time.
5. 'Pathologist Charged in Plastination Case', *Guardian*, 17 October 2002, at http://www.guardian.co.uk/world/2002/oct/17/russia.arts [accessed 28 April 2013].
6. *Independent*, 5 January 2011, at www.independent.co.uk/arts-entertainment/art/news [accessed 28 April 2013].
7. T. Marshall, *Stolen Hearts: Fiction and the 1990s' Pathology Scandal* (Nottingham: Critical, Cultural and Communications Press, 2009), p. 16.
8. Ibid.
9. *Independent*, 17 March 1999.
10. I. S. D. Roberts et al., Could Post-Mortem Imaging be an Alternative to Autopsy in the Diagnosis of Adult Deaths? A Validation Study', *Lancet*, 379 (2012), pp. 136–42.
11. R. D. Start et al., 'Clinical Necropsy Rates during the 1980s: The Continued Decline', *Journal of Pathology*, 171 (1993), pp. 63–5; H. Rickard and M. Willis, 'After Alder Hey … Can We Survive?', *Association of Clinical Pathologists News* (Summer 2001), pp. 11–13; Royal College of Pathologists, *Guidelines for the Retention of Tissues and Organs at Post-Mortem Examination* (London: Royal College of Pathologists, 2000).

Conclusion

1. *Edinburgh Medical and Surgical Journal*, 64 (1845), p. 255.
2. *Lancet*, 1 (30 May 1896), p. 1539.
3. Ibid.
4. *Lancet*, 2 (24 July 1880), p. 143.
5. Burney, *Bodies of Evidence*, p. 105.
6. *Lancet*, 1 (19 June 1909), p. 1786.
7. *USA Today*, 27 April 2006, p. 1.
8. I. S. D. Roberts et al., The Non-Invasive Post-Mortem or Minimally Invasive Autopsy', in J. Underwood and M. Pignatelli (eds), *Recent Advances in Histopathology*, vol. 22 (London: Royal Society of Medicine Press, 2007), pp. 181–98.

WORKS CITED

Primary Sources

Acts and Parliamentary Papers

2 & 3 Gul. IV c. 75: An Act for Regulating Schools of Anatomy, 1832
Hansard
Papers from the Select Committee on Anatomy
Royal Commission Appointed to Inquire into the Medical Acts, 1882
Royal Commission on Medical Education, 1836
Select Committee on Medical Education, 1834

Manuscript Sources

Bodleian Library
    MS Acland – Papers and Correspondence of Henry Acland
    MS Dep. b. 48 – Oxon Lent Assizes 1832
    MSS.Top.Oxon.c.272 and d.245 – Oxford Board of Health
Christ Church College, Oxford
    MS Estates – Anatomy School
    Visitations of Dr Lee's Anatomy School
Corpus Christi College, Oxford
    MS.263 folio 128 – Diary of Bryan Twynne
Manchester Central Reference Library
    M10/808 – Hulme Letters
    M327/1/2/1–11 – Withington Workhouse Deaths Register 1857–98
    M327/1/2/13, M327/2/5/1 – Withington Workhouse Register of Burials
    M9/36/1–2 Manchester Board of Health Papers 1831–3

University of Manchester, John Rylands Library

 Manchester Medical Collection – biographical files

 MMC/5/2/3/1–17 – Manchester Medical Schools

 Manchester Medical Society Minutes

 RA/1/1–4 – Owens College Archives 1870–1904

 RA/2/1 – Manchester University Archives 1880–1903

Manchester Royal Infirmary

 Minutes of Manchester Infirmary 1818

 Minutes of Weekly Board of Governors 1843–5

 Minutes of Special Medical Committee 1822–47

Oxford City Archives

 C/ENG/1/A1/2 – Botley Cemetery Register of Burials

 C/ENG/1/A7/1 – Rose Hill Cemetery Register of Burials

 C/ENG/1/A10/2 – Wolvercote Cemetery Register of Burials

 Reports of English Cemeteries and of the Oxford Sub-Committee, Letters etc., c.2.29, Minutes (1889–1915)

Oxford Record Office

 AU/PLU/A1/01–12 – Headington Board of Guardians Minute Books 1841–1900

 CPZ/15 – Otmoor Enclosure Papers

 PAR/189/8/F2/1 – All Saints Vestry Minutes

 PAR/207/2/A1/1 – St Martin Carfax Vestry Minutes 1762–1843

 QSP 1/1 & QSP 1/2 – Calendar of Prisoners 1778–1844

 W.4.1 – Oxford Board of Guardians Annual Reports

Oxford University Archives

 HA89 – Human Anatomy file

 HC/1/5 – Hebdomadal Council Papers

 'Remarks by Dr Acland on a Draft Report to Committee of Hebdomadal Council on Engineering and Medicine', 5 November 1879

National Archives

 HO 44/1, HO 83/1, HO 44/27, HO 42/6 – Home Office Records

 HO 83/1 – Anatomy Licenses

 MH 74/10, MH 74/11, MH 74/12, MH 74/13, MH 74/14, MH 74/15, MH 74/16, MH 74/36, MH 74/37, MH 74/38 – Anatomy Office Out-Letter Books

 PC1/93 – Central Board of Health Letter Book

 PC1/103 – Central Board of Health In-Letter Book

 TS 11/1031/4433 – Otmoor Enclosure Papers

Radcliffe Infirmary Records

    RI/C/1/1–21 – Board of Governors Minutes 1770–1904

    RI/1/26 – Out-Letter Books

    RI 1832 Cholera File

    RI9 B1/1–5 – Death Registers

Periodicals

BMA News

British Medical Journal

Edinburgh Medical and Surgical Journal

Guardian

Hospital

Independent

Jackson's Oxford Journal

Lancaster Gazette

Lancet

Liverpool Chronicle

London Medical Gazette

Mail Online

Manchester Guardian

Medico-Chirurgical Review

Oxford University and City Herald

Pamphleteer

Poor Man's Advocate

Times

USA Today

Voice of the People

Published Primary Sources

Acland, H. W., *Oxford and Modern Medicine, a Letter to Dr James Andrew* (Oxford and London: Henry Frowde, 1890).

Aiken, J., *Thoughts on Hospitals: With a Letter to the Author by Thomas Percival* (London: Joseph Jackson, 1771).

Alcock, T., 'An Essay on the Education and Duties of the General Practitioner in Medicine and Surgery', *Transactions of the Associated Apothecaries and Apothecary-Surgeons* (1823), pp. 1–135.

Alford, H., 'The Bristol Infirmary in my Student Days 1822–28', *Bristol Medico-Chirurgical Journal*, 8 (1890), pp. 165–91.

Anecdotes of Eminent Persons Comprising Also Many Interesting Remains of Literature and Biography with Some Original Letters of Distinguished Characters, 2 vols (London: Samuel Bagster, 1813).

[Anon.], *The Victoria University of Manchester Medical School* (Manchester: Manchester University Press, 1908).

Barnes, T., 'Proposals for Establishing in Manchester a Plan of Liberal Education, for Young Men Designed for Civil and Active Life Whether in Trade, or in Any of the Professions', *Manchester Memoirs*, 2 (1785), pp. 30–5.

Beddoes, T., *A Letter to the Right Honourable Sir Joseph Banks on the Causes and Removal of the Prevailing Discontents, Imperfections and Abuses in Medicine* (London: Richard Phillips, 1808).

Bell, J., *Letters on Professional Character and Manners: On the Education of a Surgeon and the Duties and Qualifications of a Physician* (Edinburgh: J. Moir, 1810).

Bellers, J., *An Essay Towards the Improvement of Physick in Twelve Proposals by which the Lives of Many Thousands of the Rich as well as of the Poor may be Saved Yearly* (London: J. Sowle, 1714).

Boyle, R., *Works*, 14 vols (London: W. Johnston, 1772).

Burdon-Sanderson, J. S., *The School of Medical Science in Oxford* (Oxford: Horace Hart, 1892).

Campbell, R., *The London Tradesman* (Newton Abbott: David and Charles, 1969).

Carus, C. G., *The King of Saxony's Journey through England and Scotland in the Year 1844* (London: Chapman and Hall, 1846).

Chamberlaine, W., *Tirocinium Medicum; or a Dissertation on the Duties of Youth Apprenticed to the Medical Profession* (London: privately printed, 1812).

Crosse, J. G., *Sketches of Medical Schools of Paris* (London: J. Callow, 1815).

Davies, R., *Epistle to the Reverend Dr Hales on the General State of Education in the Universities with a Particular View to the Philosophic and Medical Education, being Introductory to the Essays on the Blood* (Bath: M. Cooper, 1759).

Engels, F., *The Condition of the Working Class in England* (St Albans: Granada, 1982).

Farre, J., *An Apology for British Anatomy, and an Incitement to the Study of Morbid Anatomy* (London: Longman, 1827).

Fawdington, T., *A Case of Melanosis, with General Observations on the Pathology of this Interesting Disease* (London: Longman; Manchester: Robinson, 1826).

—, *A Catalogue Descriptive Chiefly of the Morbid Preparations Contained in the Museum of the Manchester Theatre of Anatomy and Medicine, Marsden Street, with Occasional Explanatory Remarks* (Manchester: Harrison and Crosfield, 1833).

Foster, M., *On Medical Education at Cambridge* (London: Macmillan, 1878).

Gaskell, S., 'Cholera in Manchester', *Edinburgh Medical and Surgical Journal*, 40 (1833), pp. 52–65.

Gaulter, H., *The Origins and Progress of the Malignant Cholera in Manchester* (London: Longman and Co., 1833).

Graves, J., 'On Clinical Instruction', *London Medical Gazette*, 10 (1832), pp. 402–3.

Green, J. H., *The Touchstone of Medical Reform Addressed to Sir Robert Harry Inglis Bart MP* (London: Samuel Highley, 1841).

Gregory, J., *Lectures on the Duties and Qualifications of a Physician* (London: W. Stahan and T. Cadell, 1773).

Guthrie, G., *A Letter to the Right Honorable the Secretary of State for the Home Department Containing Remarks on the Report of the Select Committee of the House of Commons on Anatomy* (London: W. Sams, 1829).

Hallifax, S., *A Sermon for the Governors of Addenbrooke's Hospital* (Cambridge: J. Archdeacon, 1771).

Harrison, E., *Remarks on the Ineffective State of the Practice of Physic in Great Britain with Proposals for its Future Regulation and Improvement* (London: R. Bickerstaffe, 1806).

Hearne, T., *Remarks and Collections*, 11 vols (Oxford: Oxford University Press, 1885–1921).

Hemming, W. D., *The Medical Student's Guide* (London: Bailliere, Tindall and Cox, 1876).

Hunter, W., *Two Introductory Lectures, Delivered by Dr William Hunter, for his Last Course of Anatomical Lectures at his Theatre in Windmill-Street* (London: J. Johnson, 1784).

Jordan, J., 'A Case of Obliteration of the Aorta', *North of England Medical and Surgical Journal*, 1 (1830), pp. 101–4.

Kay, R., *The Diary of Richard Kay, 1716–51 of Baldingstone, near Bury: A Lancashire Doctor*, ed. W. Brockbank and F. Kenworthy (Manchester: Chetham Society, 1968).

Keetley, C., *The Student's Guide to the Medical Profession* (London: Macmillan, 1878).

—, and R. Wharry, *The Student's and Junior Practitioner's Guide to the Medical Profession*, 2nd edn (London: Balliere, Tindall and Cox, 1885).

Kerrison, R. M., *An Inquiry into the Present State of the Medical Profession in England* (London: Longman and Co., 1814).

Lankester, E. R., *Second Annual Report of the Central District of Middlesex* (London, 1865).

Mann, J., *Recollections of my Early and Professional Life* (London: W. Rider and Sons, 1887).

Mitchell, G. A. G., 'Resurrection Days', *Manchester University Gazette*, 27 (1848), pp. 15–154.

Morgan, J. E., *The Victoria University: Why are There No Medical Degrees?* (Manchester: J. E. Cornish, 1881).

Muehry, A., *Observations on the Comparative State of Medicine in France, England and Germany during a Journey into these Countries in the Year 1835* (Philadelphia, PA: A. Waldie, 1838).

[Naples, J.], 'Manuscript Diary (The Diary of a Resurrectionist)', held at the Royal College of Surgeons of England, London; Evidence and Report of Select Committee on Anatomy, 1828.

'Observations on Medical Reform by a Member of the University of Oxford', *Pamphleteer*, 2 (1814), pp. 414–31.

Parkinson, J., *The Hospital Pupil; or an Essay Intended to Facilitate the Study of Medicine and Surgery in Four Letters* (London: H. D. Symonds, 1800).

Petty, W., *The Petty Papers* (New York: A. M. Kelley, 1967).

Quarrell, W. H., and W. J. C. Quarrell, *Oxford in 1710 from the Travels of Zacharias Conrad von Uffenbach* (Oxford: Basil Blackwell, 1928).

Ravenscroft, E., *The Anatomist; or Sham Doctor* (London: John Cawthorn, 1807).

Roberts, S., *The Lecturers Lectured, and the Dissectors Dissected* (Sheffield, 1834).

Sharkey, J. S., *The University of Oxford and Medical Education* (n.p., 1879).

Smith, J., *Some Memoirs of the Life of Dr Nathan Alcock* (London: Buckland and Co., 1780).

Smith, T. S., 'The Uses of the Dead to the Living', *Westminster Review*, 2 (1824), pp. 59–97.

Trial of John Eaton (Manchester: J. Pratt, 1827).

Thomas, V., *Memorials of the Malignant Cholera in Oxford 1832* (Oxford: W. Baxter, 1835).

Turner, T., *On Poisons and Suspended Animation* (Manchester, 1823).

—, *Outlines of a System of Medico-Chirurgical Education Containing Illustrations of the Application of Anatomy, Physiology and Other Sciences to the Principal Practical Points in Medicine and Surgery* (Manchester: Underwood, 1824).

—, *A Practical Treatise on the Arterial System* (London: Longman, 1825).

—, *An Address to the Inhabitants of Lancashire and of the Adjoining Counties on the Present State of the Medical Profession with Remarks on the Elementary Education of the Student, and the Best Means of its Acquirement. Intended to Shew the Practicality and Importance of Establishing a School (on a More Extended Scale) in Manchester for the Cultivation of Medical and Surgical Knowledge* (London: Longman; Manchester: Underwood, 1825).

—, *Outlines of a Course of Lectures on the Laws of Animal Life and the Application of Anatomy, Physiology and Other Sciences to the Principles and Practice of Medicine and Surgery* (Manchester, 1825).

—, *Anatomico-Chirurgical Observations on Dislocation of the Astragulus* (Worcester, 1843).

—, *Memoir of Thomas Turner Esq. FRCS FLS, by a Relative with an Introduction by the Rev. David Bell* (London: Simpkin, Marshall and Co., 1875).

Von Archenholz, J. W., *A Picture of England*, 2 vols (Dublin: P. Byrne, 1791).

Walker, G. A., *Gatherings from Grave Yards; Particularly Those of London; with a Concise History of the Modes of Interment among Different Nations from the Earliest Period. And a Detail of Dangerous and Fatal Results Produced by the Unwise and Revolting Custom of Inhuming the Dead in the Midst of the Living* (London: Longman, 1839).

Secondary Sources

Adami, J. G., *Charles White of Manchester (1728–1813) and the Arrest of Puerperal Fever* (London: Hodder and Stoughton, 1922).

Anning, S. T., 'Provincial Medical Schools in the Nineteenth Century', in F. N. L. Poynter (ed.), *The Evolution of Medical Education in Britain* (London: Pitman, 1966), pp. 121–34.

—, and K. J. Walls, *A History of the Leeds Schools of Medicine: One and a Half Centuries 1831–1981* (Leeds: Leeds University Press, 1982).

Archer, J. E., *Social Unrest and Popular Protest in England 1780–1840* (Cambridge: Cambridge University Press, 2000).

Atlay, J. B., *Sir Henry Wentworth Acland, Bart, KCB, FRS, Regius Professor of Medicine in the University of Oxford. A Memoir* (London: Smith, Elder and Co., 1903).

Bailey, B., *The Resurrection Men: A History of the Trade in Corpses* (London: Macdonald, 1991).

Ball, J. M., *The Sack-'em-up Men: An Account of the Rise and Fall of the Modern Resurrectionists* (Edinburgh and London: Oliver and Boyd, 1928).

Bennett, J. A., S. A. Johnston and A. V. Simcock, *Solomon's House in Oxford: New Finds from the First Museum* (Oxford: Museum of the History of Science, 2000).

Bill, E. G. W., *Education at Christ Church, Oxford, 1600–1800* (Oxford: Clarendon Press, 1988).

Blakely, R. L., and J. M. Harrington (eds), *Bones in the Basement: Post-Mortem Racism in Nineteenth-Century Medical Training* (Washington, DC and London: Smithsonian Institution, 1997).

Boardman, C., *Oxfordshire Sinners and Villains* (Oxford: Oxfordshire Record Office, 2004).

Bonner, T. N., *Becoming a Physician: Medical Education in Britain, France, Germany, and the United States, 1750–1945* (Oxford and New York: Oxford University Press, 1995).

Brockbank, W., *The Foundation of Provincial Medical Education in England and of the Manchester School in Particular* (Manchester: Manchester University Press, 1936).

—, *Portrait of a Hospital* (London: William Heinemann, 1952).

—, *The Honorary Medical Staff of the Manchester Royal Infirmary 1830–1948* (Manchester: Manchester University Press, 1965).

Burney, I. A., *Bodies of Evidence: Medicine and Politics of the English Inquest 1830–1926* (Baltimore, MD and London: Johns Hopkins University Press, 2000).

Burrell, S., and G. Gill, 'The Liverpool Cholera Epidemic of 1832 and Anatomical Mistrust and Civil Unrest', *Journal of the History of Medicine and Allied Sciences*, 60 (2005), pp. 478–98.

Butler, S. V. F., 'Science and the Education of Doctors in the Nineteenth Century: A Study of British Medical Schools with Particular Reference to the Uses and Development of Physiology' (PhD thesis, University of Manchester Institute of Science and Technology, 1982).

Bynum, W. F., *Science and the Practice of Medicine in the Nineteenth Century* (Cambridge: Cambridge University Press, 1994).

Clark, A. (ed.), *The Life and Times of Anthony à Wood* (London: Oxford University Press, 1961).

Crossley, A., 'A History of the County of Oxford', in C. R. Elrington (ed.), *The Victoria History of the Counties of England*, vol. 4 (Oxford: Oxford University Press, 1979), pp. 74–180.

Curl, J. S., *The Victorian Celebration of Death* (Newton Abbott: David and Charles, 1972).

Davidson, M., *Medicine in Oxford: A Historical Romance* (Oxford: Basil Blackwell, 1953).

Dewhurst, K., *Willis' Oxford Casebook* (Oxford: Sandford, 1981).

Digby, A., *Making a Medical Living: Doctors and Patients in the English Market for Medicine, 1720–1911* (Cambridge: Cambridge University Press, 1994).

Donnelly, F. K., 'The Destruction of the Sheffield School of Anatomy in 1835: A Popular Response to Class Legislation', *Transactions of the Hunter Archaeological Society*, 10 (1975), pp. 167–72.

Durey, M., *The Return of the Plague: British Society and the Cholera 1831–2* (Dublin: Gill and Macmillan, 1979).

Elwood W. J., and A. F. Tuxford, *Some Manchester Doctors* (Manchester: Manchester University Press, 1984).

Engel, A. J., *From Clergyman to Don: The Rise of the Academic Profession in Nineteenth-Century Oxford* (Oxford: Clarendon Press, 1983).

Ferrari, G., 'Public Anatomy Lessons and the Carnival: The Anatomy Theatre of Bologna', *Past and Present*, 117 (1987), pp. 50–106.

Fido, M., *Body-Snatchers: A History of the Resurrectionists, 1742–1832* (London: Weidenfeld and Nicolson, 1988).

Fissell, M. E., *Patients, Power and the Poor in Eighteenth-Century Bristol* (Cambridge: Cambridge University Press, 1991).

Forbes, T. R., 'To be Dissected and Anatomized', *Journal of the History of Medicine and Allied Sciences*, 36 (1981), pp. 490–2.

Gatrell, V. A. C., *The Hanging Tree: Execution and the English People 1770–1868* (Oxford: Oxford University Press, 1994).

Geison, G. L., 'Social and Institutional Factors in the Stagnancy of English Physiology 1840–1870', *Bulletin of the History of Medicine*, 46 (1972), pp. 30–58.

Gelfand, T., 'The "Paris Manner" of Dissection: Student Anatomical Dissection in Early Eighteenth-Century Paris', *Bulletin of the History of Medicine*, 46 (1972), pp. 99–130.

Graham, M., *Images of Victorian Oxford* (Stroud: Alan Sutton, 1992).

Green, J. R., and G. Roberson, *Studies in Oxford History Chiefly in the Eighteenth Century* (Oxford: Clarendon Press, 1901).

Guerrini, A., 'Anatomists and Entrepreneurs in Early Eighteenth-Century London', *Journal of the History of Medicine and Allied Sciences*, 59 (2004), pp. 219–39.

Gunther, R. T., *Early Science in Oxford*, 3 vols (Oxford: Oxford University Press, 1925).

Haslam, F., *From Hogarth to Rowlandson: Medicine in Art in Eighteenth-Century Britain* (Liverpool: Liverpool University Press, 1996).

Hurren, E., 'Labourers are Revolting: Penalising the Poor and a Political Reaction in the Brixworth Union, Northamptonshire, 1875–1885', *Rural History*, 11 (2000), pp. 37–55.

—, 'A Pauper Dead-House: The Expansion of the Cambridge Anatomical Teaching School under the Late-Victorian Poor Law, 1870–1914', *Medical History*, 48 (2004), pp. 69–94.

Jackson, M., *New-Born Child Murder* (Manchester: Manchester University Press, 1996).

Jordan, F. W., *Life of J. Jordan, Surgeon: And an Account of the Rise and Progress of the Medical Schools in Manchester with Some Particulars of the Life of E. Stephens* (Manchester: Sherratt and Hughes, 1904).

King, L. S., and M. C. Meehan, 'The History of the Autopsy', *American Journal of Pathology*, 73 (1973), pp. 514–44.

Knox, E., 'The Body Politic: Bodysnatching, the Anatomy Act and the Poor on Tyneside', *North East Labour History Society Bulletin*, 24 (1990), pp. 19–34.

Lane, J., *The Making of the English Patient: A Guide for the Social History of Medicine* (Stroud: Sutton, 2000).

Lawrence, C., 'Incommunicable Knowledge: Science, Technology and the Clinical Art in Britain 1850–1914', *Journal of Contemporary History*, 20 (1985), pp. 503–20.

—, 'Alexander Monro Primus and the Edinburgh Manner of Anatomy', *Bulletin of the History of Medicine*, 62 (1988), pp. 193–214.

—, *Medical Theory, Surgical Practice* (London and New York: Routledge, 1992).

Lawrence, D. G., 'Resurrection and Legislation on Body-Snatching in Relation to the Anatomy Act in the Province of Quebec', *Bulletin of the History of Medicine*, 32 (1958), pp. 408–24.

Lawrence, S. C., 'Anatomy and Address: Creating Medical Gentlemen in Eighteenth-Century London', in V. Nutton and R. Porter (eds), *The History of Medical Education in Britain* (Amsterdam and Atlanta, GA: Editions Rodopi BV, 1995), pp. 199–228.

Lawrence, S. C., *Charitable Knowledge: Hospital Pupils and Practitioners in Eighteenth-Century London* (Cambridge: Cambridge University Press, 1996).

Lees, L. H., *The Solidarities of Strangers: The English Poor Laws and the People, 1700–1948* (Cambridge: Cambridge University Press, 1998).

Linebaugh, P., 'The Tyburn Riot against the Surgeons', in D. Hay, P. Linebaugh, J. Rule and E. P. Thompson (eds), *Albion's Fatal Tree: Crime and Society in Eighteenth-Century England* (Harmondsworth: Penguin, 1975), pp. 65–117.

Loudon, I., 'Medical Education and Medical Reform', in V. Nutton and R. Porter (eds), *The History of Medical Education in Britain* (Amsterdam and Atlanta, GA: Editions Rodopi BV, 1995), pp. 229–49.

MacDonald, H., *Human Remains: Dissection and its Histories* (New Haven, CT: Yale University Press, 2005).

—, *Possessing the Dead: The Artful Science of Anatomy* (Melbourne: Melbourne University Press, 2010).

MacGillivray, R., 'Body-Snatching in Ontario', *Canadian Bulletin of Medical History*, 5 (1988), pp. 51–60.

Marland, H., *Medicine and Society in Wakefield and Huddersfield 1780–1870* (Cambridge: Cambridge University Press 1987).

Marshall, T., *Murdering to Dissect: Grave-Robbing, Frankenstein and the Anatomy Literature* (Manchester: Manchester University Press, 1995).

—, *Stolen Hearts: Fiction and the 1990s' Pathology Scandal* (Nottingham: Critical, Cultural and Communications Press, 2009).

Mattick, K., R. Marshall and J. Bligh, 'Tissue Pathology in Undergraduate Medical Education: Atrophy or Evolution?', *Journal of Pathology*, 203 (2004), pp. 871–6.

Maulitz, R. C., *Morbid Appearances: The Anatomy of Pathology in the Early Nineteenth Century* (Cambridge: Cambridge University Press, 1987).

McMahon, V., 'Reading the Body: Dissection and the "Murder" of Sarah Stout, Hertfordshire, 1699', *Social History of Medicine*, 19 (2006), pp. 19–35.

McManners, J., *Death and the Enlightenment: Changing Attitudes to Death among Christians and Unbelievers in Eighteenth-Century France* (Oxford: Oxford University Press, 1981).

Midwinter, E. C., *Social Administration in Lancashire 1830–1860* (Manchester: Manchester University Press, 1969).

Moore, W., *The Knife Man: The Extraordinary Life and Times of John Hunter, Father of Modern Surgery* (London: Transworld Publishers, 2005).

Morris, R. J., *Cholera 1832: The Social History of an Epidemic* (London: Croom Helm, 1976).

Nicholson, F., 'The Literary and Philosophical Society 1781–1851', *Memoirs of the Manchester Literary and Philosophical Society*, 68 (1924), pp. 97–148.

Park, K., 'The Criminal and the Saintly Body: Autopsy and Dissection in Renaissance Italy', *Renaissance Quarterly*, 47 (1994), pp. 1–33.

Peachey, G. C., *A Memoir of William and John Hunter* (Plymouth: Brendon, 1924).

Pickstone, J. V., 'Ferriar's Fever to Kay's Cholera: Disease and Social Structure in Cottonopolis', *History of Science*, 22 (1984), pp. 400–19.

—, *Medicine in Industrial Society: A History of Hospital Development in Manchester and its Region 1752–1946* (Manchester: Manchester University Press, 1985).

Porter, R., *Bodies Politic: Disease, Death and Doctors in Britain, 1650–1901* (London: Reaktion Books, 2001).

Quinault R., and J. Stevenson (eds), *Popular Protest and Public Order: Six Studies in British History 1790–1920* (London: Allen and Unwin, 1974).

Quinn, V., and J. Prest (eds), *Dear Miss Nightingale: A Selection of Benjamin Jowett's Letters to Florence Nightingale 1860–1893* (Oxford: Clarendon Press, 1987).

Reinarz, J., 'The Age of Museum Medicine: The Rise and Fall of the Medical Museum at Birmingham's School of Medicine', *Social History of Medicine*, 18 (2005), pp. 419–37.

Richardson, R., *Death, Dissection and the Destitute* (London: Penguin, 1989).

Rickard, H., and M. Willis, 'After Alder Hey ... Can We Survive?', *Association of Clinical Pathologists News* (Summer 2001), pp. 11–13.

Risse, G. B., *Hospital Life in Enlightenment Scotland* (Cambridge: Cambridge University Press, 1986).

Robb-Smith, A. H. T., *A Short History of the Radcliffe Infirmary* (Oxford: Church Army Press for the United Oxford Hospitals, 1970).

—, 'Medical Education', in M. G. Brock and M. C. Curthoys (eds), *The History of the University of Oxford, Volume VI: Nineteenth-Century Oxford, Part 1* (Oxford: Clarendon Press, 2000), pp. 563–82.

Roberts, I. S. D., et al., 'The Non-Invasive Post-Mortem or Minimally Invasive Autopsy', in J. Underwood and M. Pignatelli (eds), *Recent Advances in Histopathology*, vol. 22 (London: Royal Society of Medicine Press, 2007), pp. 181–98.

—, et al., 'Could Post-Mortem Imaging be an Alternative to Autopsy in the Diagnosis of Adult Deaths? A Validation Study', *Lancet*, 379 (2012), pp. 136–42.

Rolleston, H. D., 'The History of Clinical Medicine (Principally of Clinical Teaching) in the British Isles', *Proceedings of the Royal Society of Medicine*, 32 (1939), pp. 1185–90.

Romano, T. M., 'Gentlemanly versus Scientific Ideals: John Burdon-Sanderson, Medical Education and the Failure of the Oxford School of Physiology', *Bulletin of the History of Medicine*, 71 (1997), pp. 224–48.

—, *Making Medicine Scientific: John Burdon-Sanderson and the Culture of Victorian Science* (Baltimore, MD: Johns Hopkins University Press, 2002).

Rosner, L., *Medical Education in the Age of Improvement* (Edinburgh: Edinburgh University Press, 1991).

Royal College of Pathologists, *Guidelines for the Retention of Tissues and Organs at Post-Mortem Examination* (London: Royal College of Pathologists, 2000).

Rudé, G., *The Crowd in History: A Study of Popular Disturbances in France and England 1730–1848* (London: Serif, 1998).

Rugg, J., 'The Origins and Progress of Cemetery Establishment in Britain', in P. C. Jupp and G. Howarth (eds), *The Changing Face of Death: Historical Accounts of Death and Disposal* (London: Macmillan, 1997), pp. 105–19.

—, 'A New Burial Form and its Meanings: Cemetery Establishment in the First Half of the Nineteenth Century', in M. Cox (ed.), *Grave Concerns: Death and Burial in England 1700–1850* (York: Council for British Archaeology, 1998), pp. 44–53.

Sappol, M., *A Traffic of Dead Bodies: Anatomy and Embodied Social Identity in Nineteenth-Century America* (Princeton, NJ and Woodstock: Princeton University Press, 2002).

Sharpe, J. A., *Judicial Punishment in England* (London: Faber, 1990).

Shultz, S. M., *Body Snatching: The Robbing of Graves for the Education of Physicians in Early Nineteenth-Century America* (Jefferson, NC and London: McFarland and Co., 1992).

Sinclair, H. M., and A. H. T. Robb-Smith, *A Short History of Anatomical Teaching in Oxford* (Oxford: Oxford University Press, 1950).

Stanley, P., *For Fear of Pain: British Surgery 1790–1850* (Amsterdam and New York: Editions Rodopi BV, 2003).

Start, R. D., et al., 'Clinical Necropsy Rates during the 1980s: The Continued Decline', *Journal of Pathology*, 171 (1993), pp. 63–5.

Stone, L., *The University in Society*, 2 vols (Princeton, NJ: Princeton University Press, 1975).

Thackray, A., 'Natural Knowledge in a Cultural Context: The Manchester Model', *American Historical Review*, 79 (1974), pp. 672–701.

Thompson, D., *The Early Chartists* (London: Macmillan, 1971).

Underhill, P. K., 'Science, Professionalism and the Development of Medical Education in England: An Historical Sociology' (PhD thesis, University of Edinburgh, 1987).

Weatherall, M., *Gentlemen, Scientists and Doctors: Medicine at Cambridge 1800–1940* (Woodbridge: Boydell Press and Cambridge University Library, 2000).

Webb, K. A., 'The Development of the Medical Profession in Manchester 1750–1860' (PhD thesis, University of Manchester, 1988).

Wise, S., *The Italian Boy: Murder and Grave-Robbery in 1830s London* (London: Jonathan Cape, 2004).

INDEX

Abernethy, John, 28, 73, 74, 76
Acland, Henry, 11, 32–3, 100, 104, 106, 109, 113–20, 124–5, 127
Agricultural Revolution, 10
Alcock, Nathan, 30
Alcock, Thomas, 24
Alder Hey Hospital (Liverpool), 135, 142
Alford, H., 56–7
Anatomy Act (1832)
    and body supply, 4–6, 139–41
    and fear of anatomization, 7–8
    and independent medical schools, 11, 89–91, 93–4, 99–102, 107–9
    introduced, 79–81
    and medical reform debate, 26–7
    and Poor Law Amendment Act, 1–2, 6–7
    and public disorder/rioting, 4, 6–7, 71–2, 83–7
    public reaction to, 81–8
    'rediscovery' of, 1
    and reputation of medical profession, 9
    and 'unclaimed' bodies, 71
    wider effects of, 141–2
Anatomy Act (1984), 133
'Anatomy Debate', 16, 23–7
Anatomy Inspectorate
    and independent medical schools, 7, 89–91, 109
    and Manchester schools, 5, 92–100, 109
and Oxford University, 100–9
Anderton, Amelia, 78
Anning, Stephen, 37
Apothecaries Act (1815), 9, 37
Apothecaries Society, 36–7, 74, 125–6
apprenticeships, 5, 9, 21, 35

Aubrey, John, 46
Austin, Alfred, 96

Bacot, John, 86–7, 103
Baillie, Matthew, 33
Balfour, Edmund, 73
Barclay-Thompson, John, 114
Bate, Elizabeth, 48
Bates, Eliza, 52
Beddoes, Thomas, 24
Bedgood, William, 52
Beecham, Goody, 51
Bellamy, J., 106
Bellers, John, 11, 27–8, 50
Bentham, Jeremy, 66
Bichat, Marie Francois Xavier, 17
Bishop, John, 66, 79
Blundell, William, 72
body supply statistics, 143–60
'Body Worlds', 133–4
bodysnatching
    and 'burking', 69, 71, 72, 78–9, 86–7
    and dissection, 2–4
    documenting of, 43–4
    and higher class cadavers, 30
    increase of, 44, 139–40
    in Manchester, 53–6
    in Oxford, 50–3
    and pauper funerals, 45, 63–5
    and rioting, 66–8
    and Select Committee on Anatomy, 72–5
    sentences for, 49, 54–5, 72
Boerhaave, Hermann, 17
Boutflower, Thomas, 93, 95
Boyle, Robert, 29–30
Bristol Royal Infirmary, 135, 142

British Medical Journal, 10, 107, 111–12, 115–16, 125–6
Brodie, Sir Benjamin, 32, 74, 75–6
Bullock, Richard, 83
Burdon-Sanderson, John, 11, 100, 112–13, 115, 118–21, 124
Burke, William, 36, 55, 66, 77–8, 134
'burking', 69, 71, 72, 78–9, 86–7
Burney, Ian, 57
Byrne, Charles, 133

Cambridge University Anatomy School, 100–4, 106–7, 109
Campbell, Robert, 23
Carlile, Richard, 66
Carus, Dr C. G., 31–2
Casaubon, Isaac, 19
Central Board of Health, 81, 82, 84
Chamberlaine, William, 24
Charity Organization Society, 88
Chartism, 6
Chatham Street School (Manchester), 93, 96–7, 100
Cheeseman, Sarah, 82
Cheselden, William, 22
cholera, 4, 6, 45, 71–2, 81–5
Chorlton, Martha, 83
Christianity, 62, 80, 133
Clark, Professor, 102
Clifton, Robert, 122
Cobbett, William, 67
Company of Barber-Surgeons, 22
contemporary anatomy teaching, 131–2
Conyers, Dr, 46
Cook, Alastair, 142
Cooper, Sir Astley, 3, 22, 25, 73–4
Crowther, Dr W. L., 13
Cursham, George, 96–8, 103

Darkin, Isaac, 47
Darwin, John, 96
Davies, Richard, 24
Davis, John, 72
Davis, Vincent, 46
Davis, William, 52
Der Spiegel, 134
Doherty, John, 55–6, 62, 84
Donnelly, F. K., 4

Drake, Henry, 67
Dumville, Arthur, 93, 95–8
Durey, Michael, 29, 85

Eaton, John, 54
Edinburgh Medical and Surgical Journal, 139
Edinburgh University, 19–20, 22, 28, 77–8, 101
Edward VI, King, 29
Elliotson, John, 57
Elwood, Willis, 36
Engels, Friedrich, 7
executed corpses, 3, 7, 43–4, 45–9, 134

Fabrici, Girolamo, 16–17
Fairclough, Jane, 72
Farre, John, 26, 57
Fawdington, Thomas, 40, 53–4, 60, 92–3, 95
Ferneley, Moses, 48–9
Fissell, Mary, 12
Ford, Daphne, 136
Foster, Michael, 100, 112, 117, 125, 127
Fuller, Richard, 46
funeral security, 62–5
Furneaux, Christopher, 46

Gaisford, Prebendary, 33
Galen, 16
Gamgee, Arthur, 122, 124
Gaulter, Dr, 83
Gelfand, Toby, 17
General Medical Council, 5, 111, 121, 128–9
Gill, Geoffrey, 4
Gilpin, Mr, 55–6
Grainger, Richard, 75
Graves, Robert, 26
Green, Ann, 46
Green, Joseph Henry, 20, 74–5
Green, Philip, 67
Grosvenor, John, 31
Guardian, 134
Guide for Gentlemen Studying Medicine at the University of Edinburgh, 20
Gull, Sir William, 118
Guthrie, George, 25, 75–6

Halford, Sir Henry, 19
Hare, William, 36, 55, 66, 78, 134
Harrison, Edward, 24
Harvard Medical School, 11
Harvey, William, 19
Hawkins, Sir John, 49
Hearne, Thomas, 43, 46, 50–1
Hebdomadal Council (Oxford), 115–16,
    120
Hey, William, 22
'high style' of dissection, 17, 31
Hine, Thomas, 50
Home, James William, 55
hospital body supply, 11–13, 56–61
hospital medical schools, 27–9, 34–40,
    111–12, 124–9
HTA (Human Tissue Authority), 132
Humphrey, George Murray, 100, 103–4,
    106, 108, 116–17, 126
Hunt, Henry, 80
Hunter, John, 21, 65, 76, 95, 134
Hunter, William, 22–3, 27–8, 30, 33, 49,
    134
Hurren, Elizabeth, 5, 44, 100
Hutton, Dr Frederick, 54

Independent, 134
independent medical schools
    and Anatomy Inspectorate, 89–91, 109
    decline of, 11, 89, 90–2
    growth of, 22–3
    in Manchester, 35–40, 92–100, 109
    and Oxford University, 100–9
    pupil statistics, 161
    and Royal College of Surgeons, 5, 89–90,
        92, 109
Inglis, Sir Robert, 79–80

Jackson's Oxford Journal, 43, 47, 62, 85
Jacob, Amey, 47
Jordan, Joseph, 35–7, 39, 49, 53–4, 72, 92–5
Jowett, Benjamin, 119–20

Kay, Richard, 21
Kerrison, Robert Masters, 34
Kidd, Dr John, 31–2, 53, 82, 102–4
Knapp, Richard, 52
Knox, Dr Robert, 36, 53, 55, 134

Lamb, Richard, 47, 61
Lancet, 10, 26–7, 33–4, 61, 77, 91–2, 141–2
Lankester, Edwin Ray, 115, 117, 120–1
Lavater, D., 30
Lawrence, Christopher, 10, 18, 50
Lawrence, Susan, 9
Lawrence, William, 73
Lee, Matthew, 30–1, 48
Leeds Anatomy School, 99
Lennox, Lord William, 79
Liddell, H. G., 106, 119–21
Literary and Philosophical Society, 3, 35–6
Liverpool Mercury, 85
London Medical Gazette, 24, 26, 38, 77–8
London Medical Society, 61–2
London Ophthalmic Hospital, 26
'low style' of dissection, 17
Lower, Richard, 29–30
Luddism, 6

Macalister, Alexander, 106–7
Macalister, Donald, 119
McKeand, Alexander, 48
McKeand, Michael, 48
Macdonald, Helen, 2, 13, 44, 57–8
Manchester anatomy schools, 35–40,
    92–100
Manchester Guardian, 36, 43, 53–5, 64,
    83–4, 97
Manchester Poor Law Guardians, 7
Manchester Royal Infirmary, 13, 38, 40, 94,
    123, 127
Mann, John, *Recollections*, 57
Marland, Hilary, 58
Marsden Street School (Manchester), 92–3,
    95
Marshall, Tim, 2
    Stolen Hearts: Fiction and the 1990s'
    Pathology Scandal, 135
Matthews, William, 52
Maulitz, Russell, 57
medical education
    and 'Anatomy Debate', 16, 23–7
    and apprenticeships, 5, 9, 21, 35
    and dominance of anatomy, 16–18, 112
    evolution of, 8–11
    and hospital medical schools, 27–9,
        34–40, 111–12, 124–9

and independent medical schools, 22–3,
    35–40
and lectures, 30–2
and Manchester anatomy study, 121–4,
    127–9
and medical reform debate, 23–7
and Oxford University anatomy study,
    113–21, 127–8
and qualifications, 21, 29, 33–4
and status of physicians, 18–20
and status of surgeons, 18–19, 20–2
Medical Reform Act (1858), 121, 127
Medical Register (1858), 9
Medico-Chirurgical Review, 25
midwifery, 19
minute anatomy, 15, 41
Mitchell, G. A. G., 53
Monro *primus*, Alexander, 20, 49–50
Monro *secundus*, Alexander, 20, 50
Morgagni, Giovanni Battista, *De Sedibus et
    Causis Morborum*, 17
Morgan, John, 123, 127
Morning Herald, 66
Mount Street School (Manchester), 92
Muehry, Adolph, 31
Murder Act (1752), 3, 43–4, 45–8

Newton, Thomas, 66
Nicholls, Albert, 105
Nicholls, Frank, 30
Nightingale, Florence, 118
Novosylow, Vladimir, 134

Ogle, Professor James, 32, 118, 125
Oldham, Robert, 84
organ retention scandals, 135–6
Owens College (Manchester), 90, 99–100,
    109, 121–4, 129
Oxford Anatomy School, 3, 5, 7, 48, 105–8
Oxford University and City Herald, 66–7, 78
Oxford University Gazette, 116

Paget, George, 122–3, 126
Paget, Sir James, 118
Pamphleteer, 33
'Paris model' of dissection, 17–18, 23, 49
Parkinson, James, 24
Parsons, Dr John, 31
pauper funerals, 45, 63–5
Pegge, Sir Christopher, 52

Pelham, Cresset, 79
Penkethman, William, 54
Percival, Thomas, 28
Petty, William, 46
Phillips, J. L., 40
physicians, 18–20, 23–7
physiology, 10–11, 27, 36–9, 112–13,
    115–16, 118–20, 124
Pickstone, John, 6
Pine Street School (Manchester), 92–3,
    94–7, 100, 122
plastination, 133–4
Poor Law Amendment Act (1834), 1–2,
    6–7
Poor Man's Advocate, 55, 81, 84
Porter, Roy, *Bodies Politic*, 6
private anatomy schools *see* independent
    medical schools
private cemetery companies, 8
public attitudes to dissection, 61–8

'quacks', 2, 8, 24, 139
Quinault, Roland, 6

Radcliffe Infirmary (Oxford)
    and body supply, 7
    control of dissection activity, 41–2,
        59–60, 91, 104–5
    decline of, 125
    established, 11, 34
    influence of clergy, 41–2, 59–60
    medical education at, 115, 118, 120, 128
    post-mortems at, 13, 126, 163–4
Ravenscroft, Edward, *The Anatomist*, 65
Reform Act (1832), 36
Reinarz, Jonathan, 56
Retained Organ Commission, 132
Richardson, Ruth, 1, 5, 6, 58, 62–3, 71, 81
    Death, Dissection and the Destitute, 2
rioting, 4, 6, 45, 66–8, 71–2, 83–7
Robb-Smith, Alexander, 124
Roberts, Ian, 136
Roberts, Samuel, 86–7
Roberts, William, 91
Robinson, William, 48
Rolleston, Professor George, 100, 104–6,
    109, 114–15, 117–18
Roscoe, H. E., 122
Rosner, Lisa, 49

Rowlandson, Thomas, *The Persevering Surgeon*, 65
Royal College of Surgeons
  and hospital medical schools, 126, 128
  and independent medical schools, 5, 89–90, 92, 109
  and Manchester Anatomy School, 36, 38–40, 42
  and qualifications for surgeons, 21
  and Select Committee on Anatomy, 73, 77
Rudé, George, 4
Russell, Lord John, 101
Rutherford, Alcock, 103

Sandilands, Dr, 51
Scholefield, Reverend J., 63
'scientific' medicine, 15
Scott, Jane, 48
Sean Burrell, 4
Select Committee on Anatomy (1928), 37, 44, 69, 71, 72–8
Sharkey, John Seymour, 116
Sharp, John, 94
Shippen, William, 21
Sizonenko, Alexander, 133
Smith, Thomas Southwood, 25
  The Use of the Dead to the Living, 73
Society of Apothecaries, 36–7, 74, 125–6
Somerville, James, 85, 90–2, 93–4, 101, 102–3
Southam, George, 93, 95, 97, 122
specialist sources, 13–14
Stephens, Edward, 94
Stevenson, John, 6
Stone, Robert, 82
Suddeutsche Zietung, 133
surgeons
  and medical reform debate, 24–7
  and private anatomy schools, 22–3
  and qualifications, 21–2
  status of, 10, 18–19, 20–2
Swing Riots, 6, 66–8

Tate, Mr, 47, 61
The Medical Student's Guide, 123, 125
The Voice of the People, 78

Thomas, Reverend Vaughan, 67
Thompson, Dorothy, *The Early Chartists*, 87
Thompson, E. P., *The Making of the English Working Class*, 2
Thomson, Arthur, 100, 105, 107–9, 118, 120–1
Thorn, Edward, 47
Times, 65–6
Turner, Thomas, 25, 35–9, 53, 75–6, 90, 92–7, 109
Tuxford, Felicite, 36
Twynne, Bryan, 31

'unclaimed' bodies, 4, 71, 77
USA Today, 142

van Velzen, Professor Dick, 135, 142
Vesalius, Andreas, *De Humani Corporus Fabrica*, 16
Victoria University (Manchester), 123–4
von Hagens, Gunther, 133–4
von Uffenbach, Zacharias Conrad, 30, 50

Wakley, Thomas, 26–7, 38–9, 66, 73, 77
Walker, G. A., 63
Warburton, Henry, 73, 75, 79
Warren, T. H., 121
Watson, John, 37, 74
Weatherall, Mark, 5
West, Samuel, 118
White, Bill, 51–2
White, Charles, 35
Whittle, Glynn, 125
Why are You Afraid of the Cholera?, 82
Williams, John, 102
Williams, Thomas, 66, 79
Williamson, Mary, 60–1
Willis, Thomas, 29–30, 46
  Cerebri Anatome, 29
workhouses
  and body supply, 90–1, 94–9, 101–9, 141–2
  disorder at, 7
  and public reaction to Anatomy Act, 81
  and 'unclaimed' bodies, 4, 71
Worshipful Company of Apothecaries, 21
Wren, Christopher, 29–30

Milton Keynes UK
Ingram Content Group UK Ltd.
UKHW031149141024
449569UK00024B/940